The Rocking Chair Exercise Book

Dr. Henry F. Ogle

The Rocking Chair Exercise Book.

First published in 2010.

Printed in the United States of America.

Edited by:

Dr. Jeannine Therese Ogle
Michelle Ogle
Aleksandra Chyla
Victor Mata

Illustrations by:

Aleksandra Chyla

A very special thanks to:

All our friends and family whose love and support made this book possible.

Table of Contents

Chapter 1

Front Porch Memories

Many years ago, I stopped for a few items at a Ma and Pa grocery store in the state of Georgia. While exiting the store, I noticed a house nearby that had a long front porch. There were eight people sitting on the porch, four sitting on the porch deck and four sitting on rocking chairs. What really caught my attention was that all four of the people sitting on the deck were obese, while the four people sitting on the rocking chairs were all slim.

The porch scene remained dormant deep down in my memory until one day while I waited for breakfast outside a country restaurant. I was sitting on one of the rocking chairs in front of that restaurant and quietly bemoaning my lack of proper physical conditioning. I was locked into a busy medical practice that kept me working half-days (twelve hours a day) six days a week. Going from playing basketball five or six days a week to seldom having time for a walk had turned my six-pack abdominal muscles into a sixty-pack.

A six-pack is a term applied to two external muscles in the abdominal area, the left and right rectus abdominis muscles. The origin of these muscles is in the pubic area and they are attached at the top to the ensiform cartilage and the 5th, 6th, and 7th ribs. Each of these abdominal muscles has three transverse furrows, which, with some imagination when they're contracted, could be described as resembling a sixpack of soda pop or beer.

The goal of a lot of exercise enthusiasts is to get rid of the flab around their middle body muscles and continue working their abdominal muscles until their rectus abdominous muscles resemble a six-pack.

Moving Less and Less: Over the years I noticed the less I moved the more my physical conditioning deteriorated. I was really getting into shape, if you can call pumpkin-shaped a shape. In the old days, I had a friend who used to go on African safaris. When a group of us would go on hikes, I was the only one in our group that could walk fast enough to keep up with him. Years later, while I was waiting for breakfast at the country restaurant, I suddenly realized that I had to struggle to keep up with two-year-old toddlers.

Looking For a Solution: Frustrated with my lack of physical conditioning, I was thinking about possible solutions while I was waiting for the hostess to call my name. I realized I had to do something that I could work into my lifestyle since I wasn't in a position to retire or to walk away from my practice. As I rocked I started noticing a slight movement in my abdominal muscles. I didn't stand up and yell, "Eureka, I have found it" but it took me back to the porch scene in Georgia. Suddenly, the significance of that porch scene in Georgia dawned on me. The four obese people sitting on the porch deck were what we now call 'couch potatoes' while the four people on the rocking chairs 'kept moving.' All eight people probably started out at about normal weight, but the years of 'just sitting' or 'keep moving' probably made the difference.

An Easy Decision: Keep moving and gradually lose the extra pounds and inches or remain a couch potato and gain some more excess baggage? Rocking Chair Exercises may be an easy way to make the difference.

Keep Moving: The concept of 'keep moving' made a lot of sense to me. I discussed the keep-moving concept with one of my patients. He told me his aunt has no seats in her living room except rocking chairs and doesn't want any other seats. She was, at that time, over eighty years young, trim and going strong.

Another example of this concept I remember from my teenage years. This was an incident involving one of my adult neighbors I don't recall his name but he was retired and about 70 years old. The 70-year-old neighbor was small in stature, slim but very wiry and strong. I could see him almost every day actively moving about and working in what looked like a half-acre garden. One day a big, young punk accosted him. The punk trespassed onto my neighbor's property and started rough housing him. My neighbor was no youngster but he beat the tar out of the young punk.

People Are Less Physically Active: People were more physically active in the old days before the automobile became affordable. The adults and kids walked a lot, danced, rode bikes or scooters, played stickball or baseball, skated, played hopscotch, etc. In general, the adults and kids were physically active enough to burn off the calories.

Along came the radio, which offered only a few programs, but the novelty of it had people spending their evenings sitting and listening instead of moving about. The radio didn't have a record or rewind capability so no one dared to move or else they might miss some of the program. Many of the very early radio programs were broadcast live and were not recorded to save for future broadcasting.

Then people began to watch television. This gradually led to the death of many of the amusement parks, the dance halls with the big bands, and many more of the places and activities that provided a lot of exercise for people.

Moving Less and Getting Bigger: People are moving less and less and getting bigger and bigger. One sign of this negative change is the proliferation of extra-size clothing stores. We have a weight and physical conditioning tsunami on our hands.

Look To The Future: Late one afternoon I sat at a table in the food court of a local shopping center and watched the people passing by. Some of the young people passing by were wearing outfits with bare midriffs, that is, you could see from one to three inches (sometimes more) of their waistline sticking out between the bottoms of their shirts and the tops of their jeans or slacks. It became obvious the young people of today need a lot of waistline help. The average and overweight people, with few exceptions, had noticeable bulging at their waistlines. Many of the slim people, while looking quite trim, also had a little tummy bulging (referred to as skinny fat). Very few of the young people looked trim or physically conditioned at the waistline. It used to be that very few young people would develop a such a spread (big bottom) and/or saddle bags (pouches of fat hanging off the sides of the thighs) until they'd been out of high school for a few years and were no longer required to exercise. Now we see the spread and saddle bags developing in preschool children. They sit, sit, sit, and have little or no exercise. Some schools are trying to eliminate physical education classes so they can get more academic time. Brain cells need blood flow

and this requires exercise. Lack of exercise is a disaster that is backfiring both academically and physically. Fat cells developed in childhood are hard to beat. Sadly, many of these children never have a chance to develop their naturally healthy body shape.

Less Calories Being Burned: In 1958, the Food and Nutrition Board of The National Academy of Sciences issued recommended calorie intakes for the 'reference' man and woman. The recommendation for reference man, 5' 9", 154 pounds, 25 years old, was 3,200 calories. The recommendation for reference woman, 5'4", 128 pounds, age 25, was 2,300 calories a day. In 1964 the board reduced the recommended calories for men to 2,900 and 2,100 for women. The American Way was fast becoming the Sedentary Way. The board foresaw the truth; the average American would no longer be physically active enough to burn off the higher calorie intake. The calorie recommendations are constantly being adjusted but the truth remains - most people aren't physically active enough to burn off as many calories.

Basic Exercises: Having observed the effects of the rocking chair movements on my abdominal muscles, I started taking notes and developing some basic exercises that I felt I could do without over-stressing myself. I visited that country restaurant and their rocking chairs quite a few times in the next several months and then asked my family for my own rocking chair for Father's Day. They bought one and I started a routine of Basic Rocking Chair Exercising: about five minutes in the morning before breakfast and about twenty minutes in the evening while I watched the late evening news.

<u>My Personal Results</u>: I started observing the effects of the Basic Rocking Chair Exercises on my own body. I had only two very short workouts each day but I started to see results:

*** An inch melted off my gut in one week of one five-minute session and one twenty-minute session each day doing Basic Rocking Chair Exercises. Another four inches melted off within the next six months.**

*** The muscles in my abdomen and the front of my thighs became stronger thereby making getting out of chairs and vehicles a lot easier.**

*** My sixty-pack abdominals went down to about a twenty-four pack in about six months.**

*** My shirts fitted tighter around my chest and shoulders and draped more respectively around my waistline. It stopped looking like the lower part of my shirts had been casualties of the Battle of the Bulge.**

*** I could now see my shoes, one black, and one charcoal gray. That's funny I have a pair like this in my room.**

*** My formerly athletic abdominal muscles, which had turned to rocks of jelly, now started to show some definition instead of looking like a big soft pillow. * I noticed a definite increase in the strength of my abdominal and low back muscles and especially a reduction in that low back 'rusty hinge' feeling. * My energy increased and I started to do a few chores around the house. I noticed a significant increase in my overall strength. Three months after starting the program I was able to easily move a queen size box spring and mattress. A year earlier, I needed help to move those clumsy and fairly heavy items.**

*** A knee and an ankle that had become relatively stiff as a result of repeated sports sprains were now more limber.**

* **My family started seeing and commenting on the difference in my energy, strength, and appearance. Additionally, after they saw the shrinkage around my middle, I sometimes had to wait my turn to use my rocking chair.**

Chapter 2

Can You Make A Rocking Chair Work?

If I asked an average person to do thirty abdominal crunches (shortened sit-ups) they'd probably give me a dirty look and walk away from me in a hurry. If, however, I asked them to sit in a rocking chair and rock for one minute they'd probably think nothing of it and may actually enjoy doing it. The average rocking chair can be rocked approximately thirty times a minute. If you rocked for one minute you'd be doing about thirty modified abdominal crunches with virtually no effort and without breaking a sweat. Try it - you may like it and be totally amazed. You may be shocked at the amount of middle body exercise you can get in a rocking chair and also how painfully sore your abdominal muscles, low back muscles, thigh muscles, and buns (buttocks) can quickly become if you overdo it. I asked a teenage girl to try some Basic Rocking Chair Exercises and she had to quit rocking in less than three minutes because her abdominal muscles started hurting. You should, as with any new exercise, proceed cautiously until you're accustomed to the demands of the exercise.

I started developing basic exercises that could be performed using a standard rocking chair. My idea was that if a person can make a rocking chair work, they could do the easy exercises. People who can't do even one regular abdominal crunch may find they can easily do thirty or perhaps hundreds of modified abdominal crunches while sitting on a rocking chair. The secret is that the person is in a seated position; their body is already in a semi-crunched position, and the rocking chair supports the weight of the body thereby allowing the targeting of the abdominals,

hips, thighs, and buns. An added bonus is that middle body strength and stamina are keys to developing better upper body and lower body strength and stamina.

Rocking Chair Exercising: Imagine a doctor telling a couch potato to get into a regular program of abdominal crunches, calisthenics, walking, weight training, etc. The couch potato will usually make a significant change - to a different doctor.

I originally saw Rocking Chair Exercising as a way to gently work my own formerly athletic abdominal and low back muscles into a reasonable physical condition. I then started to visualize the exercises as a way to work the abdominal and back muscles of my patients to help stabilize their painful lower back related conditions. In business, you must always consider your target audience. My original target audience was people who were hurting structurally, that is, they were suffering from muscle spasms, muscle strains, ligament sprains, and/or herniated cartilage problems in their lower back or hip(s). My primary target audience was a large number of patients who, with help, may have spent fifteen minutes or more getting out of bed and were too rigid with muscle tightness to even take a step or even a deep breath. They may have been advised to do abdominal crunches, leg lifts, etc. This advice, however, was ridiculous. Normally all they could do was try to figure out how to deal with their pain, how to take the next step, and how to make a trip to the bathroom.

Strenuous Exercise: Strenuous workouts aren't necessary to lose weight and improve fitness. In fact, strenuous exercise is not at all essential for better health. Strenuous exercise often leads to over-use conditions such as carpal tunnel syndrome and/or tennis elbow. The best results are obtained with consistent light exercise. There are exceptions where strenuous exercise is desired due to the type of work the person performs. A concrete laborer, for example, may be expected to lift objects

that weigh 200 plus pounds. In the case of people like concrete laborers, specific and strenuous exercises may be well advised.

Muscle Contraction and Relaxation: The function of muscles is to contract. Rocking Chair Exercises create conditions where the muscles are only contracted for a very short period of time and then relax. Alternating the use of opposing muscle groups, such as the upper arm muscles, the biceps brachia and triceps brachia, allows for a more balanced flow of blood to exit and reenter the muscles, thereby improving strength, stamina, and balance.

Too much weight or resistance creates muscle tension and a quick tiring of the muscles. Lightweight repetitions help provide a balance between the contraction and relaxation of muscles and a slower buildup of lactic acid. Many physical trainers prefer and get better results using more repetitions of lighter weights, instead of using heavier weights.

Rocking chairs in serious exercise programs? I gradually became intrigued with the possibilities of using a rocking chair as a serious piece of exercise equipment. I realized that this was a way to help tens of millions of people, who were unmotivated or just physically incapable of doing a lot of other exercise.

These exercises can also help another group of people, like myself, who are too busy to exercise. This includes a lot of people like business owners, doctors, chief executive officers, presidents, etc., who are locked into 12 hour days with very little time to breathe. Pain never takes a holiday so many people in the medical professions have little opportunity to properly exercise. Many people don't have the time, energy, and motivation to stop off at a local health club to get a good workout.

A lot of people in this situation don't think of exercising. Their idea of quality time is to get a much-needed restful nap.

Sequence of Exercises: The exercises in this book are arranged to give essential exercise to the most important body areas first. Most people have some kind of time limits or constraints that restrict the time available for exercise. They may also have difficulties due to lack of energy or stamina. We address the most important exercises first.

Patients Got Involved: I started recommending the Rocking Chair Exercises to a select group of patients and they started reporting back with considerable enthusiasm. These are some of their results:

*** Loss of some or all of the excess fat around their thighs and hips.**

*** Buns lifting up and becoming firmer.**

*** Women's breasts started lifting up.**

*** Men's pectoral muscles (on the chest) became more defined.**

*** Loss of excess fat around the middle (core) muscle area.**

Rocking Chair Exercises really rock the middle body (core) muscles. There is, however, a lot of confusion about the definition of core muscles. One of my women patients has her own definition of core muscles: "I've had three kids - core muscles are something I don't have."

The dictionary definitions of core are:

1. **The central or innermost part of a thing.**
2. **The heart, as of an apple or pear, containing the seeds.**

In this writing core muscles are defined as all the muscles, internal and external, circumscribing the body at the level of the groin, including the reproductive muscles, and up to the level of and including the breathing diaphragm. The core area includes more than forty muscles that have their origins and/or insertions in this area. This includes but is not limited to the low back, gluteal, and hip, oblique, and abdominal muscles.

Middle Body (core) Muscles

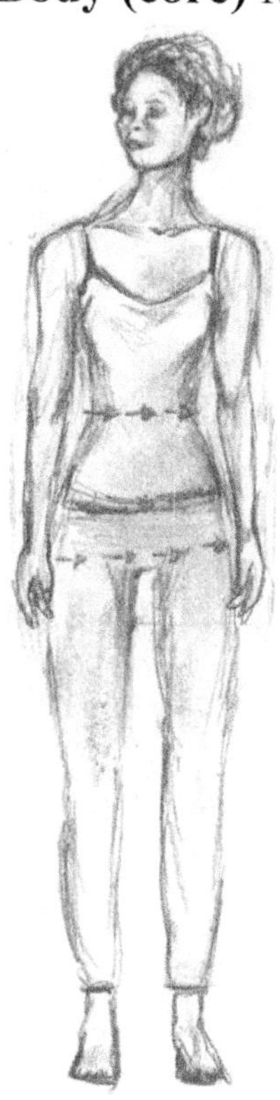

Rocking Chair Exercises stretch and tone most of the internal and external core muscles. Most people are not aware of many of these muscles. Rocking Chair Exercises work the core muscles in backward, forward, and oblique motions.

Rhythm: Each person will find they have a little different rhythm but the general rhythm is dictated by the rocking chair. Changing from one exercise or part of an exercise to another may require a temporary shift in rhythm. Words like "shift" and "reverse" will help to keep the rhythm smooth. Eventually, with regular use, the transition from one exercise to another will go pretty smoothly with either one or no skips in rhythm.

Favorite Exercise: Many people will find a favorite exercise, such as Foot wags (Exercise # 14) or Neck 45s (Exercise # 21), that really feels good or they feel the exercise is doing something positive. I find the # 4 Hands-behind-head exercises very helpful in relieving rib soreness from old sports injuries.

Feel free to do your favorite exercise(s) often but don't forget to finish your regular exercise routine. Remember to always do an even number of repetitions to keep your body balanced. You're free to pick and choose the exercises you desire. Relax and rock. Don't worry – relax, do what you can and enjoy what exercises you do. Rest anytime, do not push or overwork yourself. Relax and exercise. Some people say they never get tired of using a rocking chair.

Chapter 3

Precautions

There are some uncomfortable possibilities involved with Rocking Chair Exercises if they're improperly performed or too intensely performed before an adequate body conditioning time passes. This could result in abdominal and/or low back soreness from overused muscle fibers. The following are some general Rocking Chair Exercise guidelines:

1. See your Doctor before starting any diet or exercise program, including Rocking Chair Exercises. This is especially important for pregnant women and for people with heart problems, inguinal hernias or other hernias, diabetes, abdominal problems, and knee and/or back problems. Special attention should be given to adhesions from surgeries or injuries. If you have adhesions in your ribs or elsewhere, such as from surgery or sports injuries, the adhesions may start loosening up and get pretty sore or show up as black and blue bruises. I had a pretty significant adhesion in my left lower ribs from a sports injury that occurred over twenty years ago. I was frequently reminded of the adhesion, as it would get pretty sore. The Rocking Chair Exercises stretched out the adhesions and my skin temporarily looked like a black and blue football. It was pretty sore for a few days but hasn't bothered me since. That's a blessing. Ask your doctor about any adhesions before you start any exercise program. Your doctor may find some previously undiagnosed problem such as a heart condition or a herniated spinal disc. Body chemistry and cardiovascular health conditions may start improving

from the light exercise. People who are very subject to colds and flu may find the rocking action helps relieve some of the congested and stagnated feeling in their body. In most cases your doctor will approve of the Rocking Chair Exercise program and make additional recommendations to improve your health. People who have a tendency toward low blood sugar problems may want to start off and/or end their exercise sessions with a glass of fruit juice or whatever their doctor recommends. The substance or fluid the doctor recommends for use before and/or after exercising should help avoid the problem of going into a hypoglycemic (low blood sugar) reaction. This consideration applies to all exercises including Rocking Chair Exercises.

2. Do not eat and then do Rocking Chair Exercises. Similar to the precaution about the danger of eating and then going swimming, Rocking Chair Exercises may divert your energies away from your digestion processes and into your muscles. This could leave your food undigested and could leave you bent over with severe abdominal pain.

I had a very interesting and painful experience one Sunday afternoon. I had just eaten lunch and then proceeded to do some Rocking Chair Exercises. I did some basic exercises and then finished up by adding a few repetitions using a set of three pound weights. About an hour later I started getting severe abdominal cramps. I felt like I had a bowel obstruction and was in danger of vomiting. I almost ended up in the emergency room but it dawned on me as to what I had done. Exercising right after eating had interfered with my digestive processes and the food started rotting in my stomach and intestines. I concentrated on relieving the indigestion, relaxed for about an hour, and was okay in a few hours. Never again will I eat and do Rocking Chair Exercises. I have adopted a rule: as with swimming, do not do Rocking Chair Exercises until at least an hour after eating.

3. Fit the rocking chair to your body size. The rocking chair should be fitted to your body size. You should be able to sit with your lower back against the back of the chair. If not, use a full-length chair pad that extends from the upper shoulders to the seat of the chair. It's very important that the lower back not be at an angle such as would happen if a shorter person was sitting forward on the seat and trying to place the backs of their knees at the edge of the seat.

4. Do not sit forward on the front edge of the seat. Always sit with your lower back to the back of the seat. Sitting forward on the seat can cause a lot of stress and outright muscle soreness due to over-stressing the lower back curve. Forcing the lower back muscles into an extreme concave curve (swayback) could cause major low back muscle soreness. If necessary, use a hassock or footstool to assure your feet have something to touch. Children should use child-sized rocking chairs and not use adult rocking chairs unless the chairs are provided with a large pad. A footstool or other object should be provided for the children so their feet can touch something besides air.

5. Do not keep both of your legs outstretched in front of you while rocking; such as if you were on a swing set. It curves the lower back inward and puts a lot of pressure into the muscles of the lower back curve. This is definitely not desirable and may cause significant low back muscle soreness.

6. Do not use a lumbar support or seat that curves into or exerts pressure into the low back area. Pressure on the back should be at the level of the shoulder blades and not into the lower back curve.

7. Do only a few repetitions of each exercise until your muscles have been strengthened. The core movements use a large number of repetitions for middle body exercise in a short period of time, which could cause extreme muscle soreness

if you aren't conditioned to the exercise. For example, just five minutes of rocking would equal about 150 modified abdominal crunches, a lot of crunches for a person in poor middle body physical condition. I've had people in the test group wake up in the morning with abdominal and lower back muscle soreness. Rocking for an hour at 30 rocks a minute would mean you would have performed about 1,800 modified abdominal crunches. That could cause muscle soreness in the lower back and in the thighs and hips. Start with a few repetitions and gradually increase as your conditioning improves.

8. Remove keys, wallets, etc. from your back pockets. A common source of pain along the sciatic nerves is from having keys, wallets, or other objects in the back pockets while in a sitting position. The object may rub against or put direct pressure onto the sciatic nerve pathways causing pain, inflammation, soreness, or numbness in the buttocks and/or leg areas. This should also be kept in mind when driving or riding in vehicles.

Chapter 4

Gentle Persistence Does The Job

Some exercises and trainers approach the physical conditioning of the human being in a harsh and impatient way. In fact, the term 'no pain, no gain,' is a good example of that philosophy. A lot of people try too hard and attempt to do big things to get in shape. However, they sometimes end up hurting themselves, even causing disability by over-stretching or overworking poorly conditioned body parts. Personally, I believe in the philosophy of 'gain without pain,' that is, using gentle methods to get the person into condition without inflicting pain.

One special group that gets into a lot of trouble is the people who appear to be in good shape, that is, they're slim and appear to be trim. Slim and trim looking are not the same as being in good muscle-wise physical condition. I've seen overweight people who could easily touch their hands flat to the floor and could out-sprint almost anyone around them. I've also seen slim people who were so inflexible they could barely bend over and touch their knees.

The power is in taking little actions consistently. In the Old Testament of the Holy Bible, 1 Kings 19: 9-13, the Prophet Elijah was told "'Go outside and stand on the mountain before the Lord, the Lord will be passing by.' A strong and heavy wind was rending the mountains and crushing stones - but the Lord was not in the wind. After the wind there was an earthquake - but the Lord was not in the earthquake.

After the earthquake, there was fire - but the Lord was not in the fire. After the fire was a tiny whispering sound. When he heard this, Elijah hid his face in his cloak and went and stood at the entrance to the cave."

A lot of exercise programs are like the wind, the earthquake, and fire. I see some of the results of this in my medical practice; pain from muscle spasms, muscle strains, sprained ligaments and herniated cartilage (knees and spinal discs). For many, there's no gain, just pain.

What most people need is a gentle exercise system that slowly, safely, and effectively conditions their body parts without inflicting pain and creating disabling soft tissue (cartilage herniation and/or ligament sprain) damage. Most people need a system that can be gradually increased as they become stronger and more flexible. The starting point that's needed is a program that can bring their middle body from the couch potato stage to a more physically fit stage. The Rocking Chair Exercise program is designed to accomplish that purpose.

The Rocking Chair Exercise program makes it easy for even a couch potato to start doing an effective core muscle workout. Most of your weight is supported by the rocking chair, allowing easy movement of your middle body (core) muscles. People who can't get moving trying to do crunches on abdominal exercise devices should have no problem doing modified abdominal crunches on a rocking chair. Rocking enhances the effect of exercise. The rocking action greatly enhances the effect of the muscle activity or motion. Every rocking motion actually ends up with at least two movements, backwards and rebound. The rocking action gives a free weights effect, that is, muscles being moved and stretched in many directions. A good example of the rocking effect is when doing Exercise 39- nine pack with one weight.

Repetitions: Each exercise consists of the rocking action along with movement of certain body parts. Depending on your physical conditioning you may want to start with four repetitions and work up to ten. Always use even numbers of repetitions (4, 6, 8, 10, etc.) to keep your body muscle development balanced.

Multiplicity of Exercise Effects: The Rocking Chair Exercises rocking action automatically results in exercising many body parts. Simple rocking will affect the feet, ankles, Achilles' tendons, calves, shins, knees, inner and outer thighs, hips, buns, abdominal, obloquies, and low back. Rib exercises, for example, will affect all of the above plus the rib cage, shoulders, and upper back muscles.

Enhancing The Basic Rocking Chair Exercises: I was really impressed with the results of the Basic Rocking Chair Exercises. I then found myself adding items to enhance the effects of the exercises. I added small weights, three pounds each, which I held as I rocked. This gave a little more muscle action and resistance but did not create the boredom I usually endured doing biceps curls. I decided on doing more repetitions instead of going for heavier weights. I then added neck, chest, and leg exercises to the program and found I had a pretty good workout and all without breaking a sweat. This provided a more rounded exercise routine with virtually no effort. Beginning Rocking Chair Exercises can help to get people conditioned and to increase their energy so they may feel motivated to go on to more complete Rocking Chair Exercise routines. These people may also have fewer tendencies to get discouraged due to lack of progress or due to becoming injured or suffering severe muscle spasms.

Rocking Chair Exercise is so easy. I've seen some people who are so out of condition that they get totally pooped out just by getting into their exercise clothes. One woman told me the only way she could see what her husband looked like standing up was to lie down next to him. In my own case, my schedule during my workweek would get me home just in time to sit down, watch a little T.V., and go to sleep. Predictably, the less I did physically, the less I wanted to do, and the more weight I gained. Once I started doing the Rocking Chair Exercises the loss of one inch around my paunch in one week and another four inches in six months got me motivated to do more. With Rocking Chair Exercising, more is so convenient, comfortable, safe, and easy.

Measuring Progress: Serious exercisers may choose to measure and record their progress such as before and after measurements of range of motion (ROM). They may choose to keep track of their weight, their waist measurement, notches in their belt, or many other measurements such as hips, thighs, biceps, triceps, etc. Before and after photographs, preferably in the standing position, may be very motivating. Use the same distance, stance and same type of clothes each time you take pictures.

Chapter 5

Selecting And Maintaining A Rocking Chair

Having a rocking chair in your home and/or workplace can make Rocking Chair Exercising very convenient. If you have a lull in the action or decide to exercise at midnight or 3 A. M., whether rain, snow, sleet, heat, or cold, your exercise equipment is there for you.

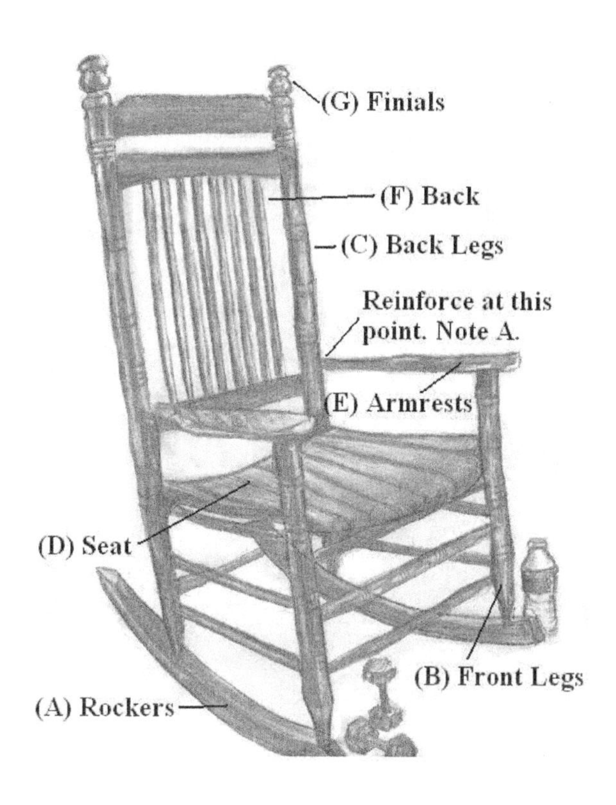

Standard Rocking Chair With Armrests And Finials

The rocking chair consists of many parts. Only a few parts are identified herein as they'll be referred to during the exercise routines. The rocking chairs consist

primarily of: two rockers or skates (A), two front legs (B), two back legs (C), a seat (D), two arms or armrests (E), a back (F), and two finials (G), which are on top of the two back legs. Note A: Make sure the Rocking Chair is reinforced where the backs of the armrests meet the uprights of the back legs. This is the most common place of separation of the parts.

<u>History</u>: Rocking chairs have been around for centuries. The invention of the rocking chair is attributed to Benjamin Franklin in the 1760s. Many of the original chairs had no back or armrests and were made from crude materials such as twigs and rough lumber. The rockers (A), the curved boards at the bottom of the rocking chairs, were referred to as skates. Rocking chairs were not considered to be good furniture as they were fairly crude. Eventually rocking chairs were built as fine pieces of furniture, became commonplace in many homes and could sell for thousands of dollars. Some rocking chairs have been sold for over $ 40,000.00. You probably don't want to use an item that valuable for Rocking Chair Exercises. Excellent rocking chairs, suitable for exercises, currently are available for less than $ 200.00.

<u>Features of Rocking Chairs</u>: There are a lot of different kinds of materials used in building rocking chairs. The frames are usually made from hardwoods such as oak or maple. Better quality chairs may be created using a combination of airdried and kiln-dried hardwoods, such as red oak, which can adjust to the different effects of heat and/or cold conditions. Some frames are made of various metals such as rolled steel.

The seats and backs are made of many different materials such as wicker, rattan, wood, wire mesh, leather, rawhide, and fine textiles.

The armrests may have different shaped front ends such as having beveled or mushroom shaped handgrips.

Comfort: It's very important to be comfortable during exercise. People will tend to exercise more consistently if the exercise apparatus is comfortable. The position of the back, the height and width of the armrests, and the height, depth, and width of the seat all work toward comfort. Rocking chairs with wood slat backs and seats may need a chair pad for comfort. The chair pad should be firm against the person's wings (scapulas) and lower back. You may need wider seats for wide people and deeper seats for long legged people.

Location: An important early decision is to determine where you want to locate the rocking chair. The rocking chair area should have a healthy air flow capability but away from drafts. Exercising under or near a ceiling fan, near an open window, or on a screened-in porch may be good choices for staying very comfortable.

1. **Indoor Setting:** You may want to have the rocking chair facing an entertainment center or a picturesque outside view. Watching TV and rocking can give you, at 30 rocks per minute, approximately 1,800 modified abdominal crunches per hour. You'll need room, approximately 20+ inches wide for a child's size, 27+ inches for an adult size, and 48+ inches for a double rocker. You'll need additional room for spreading out your arms, bird style, during exercise and this may require a total width of about six feet plus a few inches for clearance.

You may choose to have a rug or an exercise equipment mat under your rocking chair to protect against damage to the carpet or flooring.

2. Outdoor Setting: Your rocking chair should be sheltered from rain, snow, extreme heat, and extreme cold. Porches, greenhouses, and screened-in rooms are usually good choices. You may choose to provide adequate lighting. You may choose to have an exercise equipment mat or a rug to minimize 'walking', reduce noise, and protect against damage to the flooring. Make sure your rocking chair isn't too close to other rocking chairs or other objects. You'll need to allow a clear space on each side of the rocking chair to prevent finger jamming or restriction of movement while exercising. If you have multiple chairs, it may be helpful to move every other chair forward to allow adequate arm room while exercising.

Décor: Does the rocking chair match or blend with your home or business decor? Make sure your rocking chair matches or blends in. Think of the novel design possibilities. You can decorate your rocking chair for various occasions such as Christmas or Easter. You can also decorate the chair for the seasons of the year or special occasions such as birthdays.

Safety:

*** Do not rock after eating - please observe the precautions in Chapter 3.**

*** Look under the rocking chair(s) before each use.**
You may find electric wires, cats, dogs, glass, etc.

*** The rocking chair should be on a stable surface.**

*** The rocking chair must be well balanced and in good repair.**

*** Never stand on a rocking chair.**

*** How much weight can your rocking chair hold? Heavier people may need a double or a specially reinforced rocking chair.**

*** Look for nearby rocking chairs, sharp edges or other objects that could cause injuries such as jamming your fingers. Remember that rocking chairs tend to walk and your chair or another chair may close in on your fingers and jam them. * Make sure the rocking chair doesn't tip sideways or backwards.**

*** If a toddler is placed on the rocking chair, secure the child to the seat. The movement of the child and the rocker may topple the child onto the floor. * People**

with open porches may be well advised to tie the rocking chair to the balcony to avoid loss in a windstorm.

* **Rocking chairs that are situated anywhere near the end of a porch or a potential drop-off area should be fastened to the floor or wall. This will help prevent the chair from walking off the side or back and dumping the person onto the ground or into the river or whatever is near them.**

Maintaining A Rocking Chair: A rocking chair that squeaks and walks the floor usually needs balancing or some other kind of maintenance. Some floors inside homes and buildings are not balanced. The walking of the rocking chair may be due to a floor imbalance.

Rocking chairs should be reinforced at the back of the armrests where they attach to the back legs. A lot of chairs have screws that are screwed in from the rear of the back legs. These screws tend to be under a lot of stress and rocking may tear the fibers inside the wood. This may result in the chair breaking at this point. I believe the screws should be screwed in from the sides of the back legs so it gives a bracing effect instead of relying on the screws not ripping out the fibers in the armrests and back legs.

Equipment Safety Check: Safety check your rocking chair and other equipment before starting your exercises. Make sure you don't have a screw loose. A squeak is a good indication of a need for maintenance. Also check to be sure there's nothing under the chair such as a cat's tail or an electric wire. A rock or a dog bone under a rocker can give you quite a heaving shock. An occasional sweeping of the floor and cleaning of the bottom of the rockers will help assure a smoother ride.

Buying A Rocking Chair: Where can you buy rocking chairs and how much do they cost? The chairs come in three basic (approximate) sizes: children's 20 inches wide, adult 27 inches wide, and double 48 inches wide. There are many sizes in between but these may be harder to find.

I don't recommend the use of the glider type rocking chairs. Also, the rocking chair must have armrests if you want to use the chair for exercise. You should have finials at the top of the back legs to provide a future ability to do resistance cord exercises or other exercises.

Don't forget you're buying a piece of exercise equipment, not a status symbol such as a chair with fancy carvings and veneered surfaces. These features may be attractive, but may be destroyed by the stress of using the chair for exercise. You may find some rocking chairs already decorated with symbols such as a state or school name. You may have people competing to use your rocking chair so you may choose to get two or more rocking chairs. The rocking chairs should be decor compatible or complementary.

The size should be considered. Do you have petite gymnasts or basketball players? You may need a small hassock or foot-prop for people whose feet cannot reach the floor. I don't recommend buying a double size rocking chair for exercising unless a regular chair is too small. Consider the height of the seat and back, the width of the seat and the depth of the seat. Shorter people may need a shorter seat (or a thick back pad) while a very tall user may need a deeper seat. There's a pressing need for rocking chairs for large people. You may want to find a craftsman who can take your measurements and create a custom fitted rocking chair just for you. You may also want to get a color and material compatible rug for under the chair. The rug should help reduce noise and wear and tear on the floor. It should

not be so thick that it interferes with rocking. You may choose to use a rug instead of an exercise equipment mat.

Sources Of Rocking Chairs: You may have fun finding the right rocking chair for your needs. There are many possible sources:

Country Stores and Restaurants,

Furniture stores including fine furniture stores,

Antique shops,

Resale stores,

Estate and auction sales,

Garage sales and flea markets,

Catalog sales,

Internet,

Cabinet and woodworking shops, Hardware and lumber stores, and finally relatives and friends.

Be sure you tell them why you want their rocking chair. That way, they won't complain later if they choose the rocking chair exercises and may have to search for one for their own needs.

Cost: How much will a rocking chair cost? Rocking chairs can be purchased for under $ 200.00 and up to many hundreds of dollars depending on variables such as materials used, age, and history. Keep in mind you are buying an item of exercise equipment, not a fancy piece of furniture for the 'don't touch' living room.

Chapter 6

Equipment Needed

Rocking Chair Exercises, like most effective exercise programs, require some special equipment:

* Rocking chair. A regular rocking chair with armrests and finials - not a glider type rocker unless it can rock fully and easily like a regular rocking chair. Make sure it fits your body size and has armrests and finials, as they're essential to have during many of the exercises.
* Chair Pad (optional). A chair pad can be used for comfort and to properly support the person's back while they're using the rocking chair. The person should be able to sit comfortably with their upper back and lower back against the chair pad. They may want to have a chair pad if they have a wicker-backed chair and also have a cat around their house. Cats like to sharpen their claws on wicker.
* Foot Prop. Shorter people may need a footstool or something else under their feet to allow their feet to touch some solid object.
* Hand Weights - 1 to 3 pounds for women and 3 to 5 pounds for men.
* Two Soft sponge-type football shaped balls, approximately six inches long and 3 inches in diameter. The football shaped balls fit the hands the best. Squeezing the sponge balls while rocking promotes strength and flexibility of the hands, wrists, forearms, and elbows. The hand strengthening exercises should be helpful exercises for golfers, baseball players, people who participate in other sports, and for people with arthritic problems in their hands, wrists, and/or elbows.

* **Resistance Cords, bands, or tubing. The resistance items aren't needed until you start Exercise # 42.**
* **Exercise Equipment mat or a rug for use under the rocking chair (optional). The mat or rug will reduce floor noise and help to prevent damage to the floor surface. The mat or rug may also help reduce some of the chair's 'walking', a natural happening especially outdoors as most porches and many other structures are pitched lower at one end to allow for proper water drainage.**

Chapter 7

Grandma's Good Advice For You And Baby

If a young woman tells her friends that she is expecting a baby they will probably tell her about all of the new, innovative, cribs, strollers, and other interesting baby gadgets on the market. When she tells grandma, however, her grandmother will probably tell her,

"How wonderful, my dear you need a rocking chair."

Grandma is right. Using a rocking chair for exercise before and after having a baby is a very good idea.

I have a theory about using Rocking Chair Exercises to help women prepare for pregnancy, delivery, and postpartum (after childbirth). Remember, you're a mother the moment you conceive. Someone may tell you that you swallowed a watermelon seed. It may look like that later on but a watermelon doesn't have fingernails, detectable brain waves, and heartbeats nor does it learn how to kick inside you. You're blessed with one of the greatest events of your life - there's a baby growing inside you.

I discussed my rocking chair theory with several of my women patients. The discussion with one of the patients, a mother of three children, helped to key me into what I believe is a partial solution to one of the problems facing many mothers, that is, long hours in labor. My patient told me that she had a very tough time with the delivery of her first child, with labor lasting about 26 hours. She seldom used her rocking chair before her first baby was born, but after delivery she used to spend a lot of time in her rocking chair, rocking her baby to sleep or to calm him. A second child presented a relatively easy delivery with labor lasting only about four hours.

The second child is usually easier, but this was a dramatic difference. Again, the woman spent considerable time in her rocking chair, rocking her new baby. A third delivery also went relatively easy.

The key I see is that rocking her babies in her rocking chair had the woman doing hundreds or perhaps thousands of modified abdominal crunches every day. As a bonus, the weight of her baby added a certain amount of muscle resistance training. The woman could do so many modified crunches because the rocking chair supported her body weight. This allowed her to unknowingly target many of the primary muscles needed for pushing during the birthing of babies. By the woman doing so many modified abdominal crunches, the Rocking Chair Exercising helped her to burn off calories, to retighten her middle body skin, and to regain the firmness of the muscles of her tummy, thighs, and buns. Of course as with any exercise program, if you are pregnant discuss it with your doctor first. Also always be gentle and use caution, understanding how fragile your baby is. If you ever feel any pain or discomfort, stop immediately and consult your doctor.

Nodding (nutation): During pregnancy, a hormone called Relaxin kicks in and relaxes the ligaments of the pelvis (ligaments tie bone to bone) thereby allowing the pelvic joints to stretch and for the pelvis to nod. This nodding, or nutation, involves a tilting of the pelvis and a spreading of the pelvic joints.

It's not unusual for a woman to spend less time in labor with her second and subsequent babies because the tissue stretching that occurred with her first nutation normally has a residual effect. Some of the stretching of the pelvic area ligaments, muscles, and tendons remain a part of the woman's shape and this makes it easier to deliver a baby.

My Theory: My theory is that Rocking Chair Exercising may provide easy and effective ways to target groups of muscles that are involved in the birthing process. The resultant increase in middle body flexibility, strength, and stamina may, in many cases, help to significantly reduce the amount of time the woman spends in labor, the amount of pain endured by the woman while in labor, and the amount of time the baby spends in the birth canal.

Less Physically Active: In general, women of today are usually very busy but not physically active. Some are busy working at a computer (sitting) or driving back and forth (sitting) to work, church, school, shopping, etc. Some women are involved in very physical jobs such as being a waitress but these occupations, with some exceptions, normally do not provide adequate middle body exercise.

Women were much more physically active in days gone by, before the advent of modern conveniences such as the washing machine, the dishwasher, and the automobile. Add to those items the invention of the radio, the TV, video games, and the Internet and you have a populace that's sitting more and more and doing less and less physically. Some people now do their shopping on the Internet and never get the exercise they used to get when they walked the stores to shop. With some exceptions, women went through labor and recovery much faster than they do today. Women now spend long agonizing hours in labor and often end up with a Cesarean section. In general, the women of yesteryear had more muscle power in their middle bodies. They were walking, bending, stooping, sweeping, mopping, scrubbing clothes, washing dishes, chopping wood and much more. Those days may be gone forever so we need new solutions to the problems of inadequate physical activity. An hour of vigorous exercise once in a while helps but it's not enough - the activity has to be more ongoing and consistent.

Test your abdominal strength and stamina. A good test for young women is to find a regular rocking chair with armrests (not a glider rocker) and try to rock for five minutes or 150 rocks. If the woman is in unusually good middle body physical condition she may be able to rock for five minutes before her muscles give out or get painfully sore. At that point in time, if her muscles give out or get painful, she may have enough time to work on her middle body flexibility, strength, and stamina. She may have time to get into a good middle body-conditioning program, which should include Rocking Chair Exercises. Can you ask an eight-month pregnant woman to do regular abdominal crunches? Of course, not, but considering the possibility of labor contractions, with her doctor's permission, she may find she can do some modified middle body exercises using a rocking chair.

During the delivery of her baby there's no going back later to work on her middle body strength and stamina. Whatever power she has in her abdominals and other middle body muscles when she goes into labor is all she's going to have to work for her. Women should start working seriously on their middle body strength, flexibility, and stamina right away. A good regiment would be to start exercising on a rocking chair for five minutes or more, twice a day, and then add time until you reach half an hour. This can be done while watching TV.

Don't expect to be pushing constantly for hour after hour during the birthing process. The pushing normally will be on and off. Like tennis where you have bursts of intense activity and then ease up for a while, the birthing process will normally give you some chance to rest briefly between pushes.

Pregnancy And Diabetes: Some women develop Diabetes Mellitus during their pregnancy and the diabetes later clears up after the delivery. A carefully

controlled diet and regular exercise, such as Rocking Chair Exercises, may help to minimize the problems from the diabetes. Make sure your doctor monitors your salt levels before changing your salt intake habits.

Exercise is very important during pregnancy. It's very important that you follow your Doctor's advice on exercise and nutrition. Exercise helps to get you ready for the demands of the birthing process and helps to control appetite and blood sugar levels. It also helps to maintain flexibility, strength, and stamina. In addition to Rocking Chair Exercises, your doctor may prescribe specific exercise classes like Lamaze.

Breathing Exercises: Some of the most important exercises for pregnant women are the breathing exercise programs such as the Lamaze method. The classes are designed so the mother, with the help and support of the father or other supportive person, learns proper breathing and pushing techniques. These breathing techniques are thought to increase the level of the pain-reducing hormones and also help assure an easier and faster delivery. Like any other exercise program, the woman should start the training as soon as her doctor recommends and not wait until she has little time before going into labor.

Breast-Feeding: Some women cannot breast-feed or may choose not to breast-feed. If a woman can, she should definitely consider breast-feeding. Many hospitals have obstetric and pediatric staff who strongly advise and support breastfeeding. Breast-feeding, as many women have discovered, is a natural function but it must be learned. A woman doesn't just place the baby at her breast and that takes care of everything. Breast size makes very little difference in her ability to breastfeed as much of the milk supply is inside her chest, not in her breasts.

Many hospitals have staff members, sometimes referred to as Lactation Counselors, who are well trained in the science of breast-feeding and are both helpful and patient with women who choose to breast-feed. The programs offered by the hospitals usually include a general prenatal program plus a prenatal and postpartum breast-feeding program. A Lactation Counselor may be able to teach the woman how to teach 'Little Nipper' not to nip. Some hospitals have or recommend local social and support groups for breast-feeding mothers.

Many women have found that breast-feeding is usually much easier than bottle-feeding. There is no need to sterilize bottles and nipples. The breast is very convenient and the milk is normally clean, easily digestible, and always at the right temperature. The mother's immune system helps to protect the child. Breast-fed children normally experience less diarrhea, allergies, teeth problems, and infections. Relax and gently exercise while holding your baby. Whether you bottle or breastfeed, you will soon find that your rocking chair will be your favorite place to feed your baby. Very gentle Rocking Chair Exercising while holding a baby gives the woman an excellent potential for bonding with her baby. The calming effect on babies who have just been vaccinated or are teething is a special blessing, and the mother can get some middle body exercise at the same time. Please always be careful not to rock too hard. Your baby is fragile.

Rocking Music: You may want to find some wonderful and peaceful rocking chair songs to play for your baby and yourself. Music is ideal for listening to while you rock and calm a restless or teething baby or toddler. Read, talk, and sing to your baby even while your baby is in your womb. Establish peacefulness so the music and

rocking encourages the baby to be calm and happy. Save the bouncy music for later for dancing around with your child.

Most babies enjoy their mother's singing. You may think your voice sounds like asthma set to music or like a cat on the back fence but your audience is a baby who loves you. If your baby is okay with your singing, it's okay to sing. Come to think of it, this may explain some of the music that's so popular with kids today.

Your Grandmother may have some good rocking chair music for you, such as the music she used to rock your father or mother to sleep. Ask Grandmother about songs such as "Rocking My Baby to Sleep in My Old Rocking Chair" or an old cowboy song "Rock Me to Sleep In My Saddle." You may also hear some tidbits from Grandmother that you can use to blackmail your parent. Rocking, music, and feeding - what a wonderful combination for mother and baby.

Food Choices And Pregnancy: One rule is very important - do not do extended Rocking Chair Exercises for at least an hour after eating. As stated in Chapter 3, Precautions, you may end up with abdominal cramps.

Proper nutrition and exercise are essential parts of any pregnancy and postpartum program. As much as I believe in exercise being essential for good health, good nutrition must go along with the exercise. Good nutrition provides the basic materials for building and repairing every human body cell. Inadequate nutrition in the mother's diet is often a factor in babies being born less than healthy. Excellent nutrition is of paramount importance during pregnancy. Human body cells aren't made from exercise, rest, and prescription medications. Babies are made from substances from inside the father and mother plus air, water, and food substances. Other items or actions may help the body create healthy body cells but they're not basic building blocks of the body cells.

We don't know the full effects of all the well- known and heavily studied nutrients such as certain vitamins and minerals. There may be many undiscovered benefits of the little studied nutrients and these nutrients may be of extreme importance to your health and that of your baby. That's why it's so important to have a diet of whole natural foods. Researchers have traced many childhood, teen, and adult health problems to what the person was fed as a child. This includes what the mother did not eat or what she ate when the baby was in her womb.

Dietary Recommendations:

*** Fresh fruits & vegetables - vital for cell growth, healthy skin, bones, and eyes. * Protein - important in building the body cells of the new baby and rebuilding the body cells of the mother.**

*** Calcium - vital for muscle, heart, and nerve development. Inadequate calcium intake has been linked to many serious pregnancy risks including low birth weight, premature delivery, and death of the infant and/or the mother.**

Researchers claim that boosting calcium intake to 1,500 to 2,000 milligrams a day may help to avoid or reduce two of pregnancy's most serious complications: high blood pressure and Preeclampsia, a toxemia of pregnancy. Preeclampsia may lead to high blood pressure, bleeding, stroke, and possible death of the mother and baby. I have listed below some vitamins that are very helpful during pregnancy: * Vitamin C - important in the development of proper growth, strong bones, and teeth.

*** Iron - essential for the developing blood supply of the fetus and for your own expanding blood supply. Pica, a strange craving for non-food items such as clay, ashes or plaster, may have its origin in inadequate minerals, especially iron.**

* Vitamin B - important in prevention of birth defects and promoting intelligence and nervous system functioning. Deficiencies of Vitamin B are sometimes shown to be a factor in cases of a lot of morning sickness.
* Vitamin E - (d-alpha form, not dl-alpha) research shows deficiency of Vitamin E can lead to muscle wasting diseases. Research has also shown Vitamin E is essential to implanting and retaining the fertilized ovum (egg).

Stress Management: Learning to handle stress constructively is a priority during pregnancy. Take control now for a healthy and positive pregnancy.

* Get plenty of sleep to help rid the body and mind of tension and anxiety. Many women can power nap, that is, take a ten or fifteen minute nap and be back to full energy. Others need a two-hour nap. Naps should not be taken too late in the evening as they may interfere with getting a full nights sleep.
* Avoid caffeine and other stimulants as they can affect your sleep and may make you and your baby hyper.
* Exercise to help ease stress. Any form of exercise you enjoy may be helpful. Rocking Chair Exercises are highly recommended.

Benefits Of Exercises: If you followed an exercise program before pregnancy you can most likely, except with aggressive and/or contact sports, continue but with the consent of your physician. If you're using a new program, start your new program slowly and wisely. Exercise helps pregnancy in several ways:

* Enhances the transport of oxygen and nutrients to the fetus.
* Decreases the risk of varicose veins and fluid retention.
* Helps to relieve or minimize back pain.
* Builds endurance for a potentially quicker, easier delivery.

*Allows for a better physical shape after giving birth.

Exercise Precautions During Pregnancy: Exercise during pregnancy is normally of great benefit to the mother and baby. There are four significant precautions to exercising while pregnant:

1. **Overheating:** Exercising in hot conditions or working hard at exercising can cause overheating problems and negatively affect the baby. Rocking Chair Exercises, in normal room conditions, usually will not overheat the body. Stop exercising if you start getting overheated. Exercising under or near a ceiling fan may be helpful in remaining comfortably cool.
2. **Blood Being Carried Away From The Baby:** Vigorous exercise may draw blood away from your baby. Rocking Chair Exercises normally help to promote blood supply to the baby.
3. **Stress On The Joints:** The limited rocking actions of the Rocking Chair Exercises will normally promote joint mobility without stressing the joints.
4. **Posture Discomfort:** Posture discomfort should be minimized while doing Rocking Chair Exercises. This may be helpful in preparing the core muscles to be stronger and more responsive during the delivery process. Your doctor must be your guide in any exercise activities and especially if there's a problem pregnancy.

Fluids For Two: As body fluids increase during pregnancy so does your need for fluid intake. Be sure to consume plenty of clean water each day. Water can come from many sources including milk, water-rich fruits, vegetable juices, and soups. Your main source of water should be from fresh water. Caffeine intake should be

restricted. Caffeine is a diuretic and stimulates movement of fluids out of your body and may cause dehydration.

Extra fluid intake is very important. A lot of bloating with drinking water may signal a salt deficiency. They've found people who died from dehydration but had a belly full of water. Tests showed they were out of salt. Consult your doctor if you tend to get bloated on fluids.

Fluids are extremely beneficial for many reasons:

*** Reduce the risk of urinary tract infection. * Rid the body of toxins and waste product.**

*** Lessen the likelihood of constipation.**

***Reduce excessive swelling.**

*** Help keep skin soft and glowing.**

Chapter 8

Surprising Benefits Of Rocking Chair Exercises

Conditioning the core muscles can make life easier in many ways. It can make chores around the house easier. Work gets done faster with improved middle body conditioning. Lawn mowing, trimming, edging, pulling weeds, raking leaves, snow shoveling, and other jobs get done quicker and easier with the increased middle body strength and flexibility. Pulling weeds, for example, usually requires a lot of frontal thigh strength in order to get up and down and move around quickly.

Your rocking chair will eliminate excuses not to exercise. Hot, cold, rainy, or snowy weather, being alone, danger on the streets, distance to a good sports facility, etc., all contribute to people's reluctance to go somewhere to exercise. The person may have had a bad experience with an injury due to participating in a poorly conceived exercise program.

Therapy Possibilities: There may be many other applications of Rocking Chair Exercises such as when using double size rocking chairs. The double sized rocking chair may, in some instances, be adapted to help give therapy to a second person. You can sit next to someone who is in very bad shape and then rock very easily. This form of therapy can be easy on the person being treated and on the person doing the therapy. The light exercise may help to build up the physical conditioning of the person rocking with the patient. This person might be a spouse or

an adult child. This might be a lot more pleasant and get done more often than other forms of exercise.

Air Supply: Breathing exercises help increase air supply to the body and stimulate the muscle tissues and organs inside the abdominal wall. Some researchers claim that increasing fresh air intake helps to increase the amount of pain-reducing hormones and to speed up the burning of unwanted fat deposits. The best results are achieved if the person is outdoors or if they exercise near an open window. Whenever possible do your Rocking Chair Exercises or any other exercises outdoors. Rib soreness or tension is often found in people suffering from asthma, smoker's hack, emphysema, or other breathing problems. The rocking chair rib stretching exercises may be very helpful but some exercises may not be doable for some of these suffering people. Let your doctor be your guide in this matter.

Sleeplessness: It's 3 A. M. and you're restless and wide-awake. It's too late to take a sleep-aid, as you have to get up in a couple of hours. Rocking Chair Exercises, especially neck, shoulder, and rib cage exercises, may help you relax and may be effective in helping you get back to sleep. Instead of tossing and turning, doing Rocking Chair Exercises can provide both relaxation and toning of the body.

Reduce Stress: Rocking Chair Exercises may help to relieve stress. One concept in calming the mind is to do something physically active which then helps to divert the thinking process to the physical action. Exercise of any form helps to move the blood and lymph, pumping out the nerve-irritating life-threatening toxins and bringing in the health building nutrients. The glands of internal secretion, especially the adrenals, may also benefit from the muscle action stimulating movement of the fluids in the body.

Pump Blood And Energy: Blood is the great healer. Keeping circulation moving to an area of the body helps to make that part more resistant to disease. It's easier for disease to set in if anybody area is stagnant. Exercise helps to move nutrients, such as calcium, into the muscles and bones. It also helps to move joint health nutrients, such as glucosamine and water, into the tissues of the joints. In tests with baseball pitchers' researchers found that a player's pitching arm invariably has stronger bones with more bone density. Rocking Chair Exercises should help improve nutrient movement into the bones and joints, especially in the middle and lower body areas, and help to improve the health of these body parts.

Elimination Of Toxins From The Body: Exercising the body with Rocking Chair Exercises may help stimulate the elimination of bodily wastes through the respiratory system, kidneys, and bowels. The exercises may also help to stimulate the lymph system. The lymph system contains a whitish fluid that moves nutrients in and toxins out of major body parts. Keeping the blood and lymph moving are basic requirements for maintaining health.

Exercise Without Dehydration Problems: Dehydration problems that often occur with other exercise routines, are minimized, as few people will actually sweat while doing Rocking Chair Exercises.

Better Cholesterol Levels: People trying to control their cholesterol levels will normally find that exercises, including Rocking Chair Exercises, help to increase the

levels of the HDLs (high density lipids) and reduce the levels of LDLs (low density lipids). Exercise normally has a very positive effect on cholesterol levels and ratios.

Work Off Excess Energy: People, such as children, who are jittery or antsy may benefit from Rocking Chair Exercises. Getting them to rock may give them an outlet for working off excess energy or tension.

Weight Control: One of the concepts I try to instill into my patient's minds is that there's often a relationship between the cell integrity of their body structures and weight problems. Aging or deterioration of the tissues due to lack of exercise and/or inadequate nutrients really raises havoc in and about the body joints. Many desire to exercise and try to exercise but structural pain cuts them down. Injuries from sports or other activities often leave persistent knee pains or other pains that may be relieved a bit by sitting down. This may help with pain control but sitting down a lot usually results in weight gain. Keeping your weight under control normally requires that you 'keep moving.'

You should exercise for strength and agility but should avoid those activities that threaten to cause structural injuries. Leave tackle football and octogenarian rugby to people who choose to endanger their future structural health and appearance. Look around and witness the dilemma of many former athletes who now have difficulty walking due to knee pains or other structural pains. Notice also that most of them have gained a lot of weight.

Rocking Chair Exercises and many other exercises help to exercise the knees and other joints. However, getting adequate nutrition into the body cells and preventing joint injuries are also important. The exercises are important to the process as exercise helps to bring the nutrients into the joints and other body tissues. Middle body muscle imbalance is also a big problem. Little actions like walking on a beach

with one foot in the water and one foot on the sand can disturb your middle body balance. This places extra joint stress on the joints on one side of your body. Imbalanced middle body problems will tend to tire a person quicker and then, what do most people do? They get tired so they sit down and gain weight. Then carrying the extra weight makes them tire easily so they sit down more often and gain more weight.

Target the structural integrity problems first and then the weight. Enjoy balanced and healthy joint integrity as nature intended. Keep moving. What do contractors do when they start rehabilitating a building? They do roof and foundation repairs first. Your hips, knees, and several other body structures are your foundation. What can you do?

1. Address any middle body imbalance problems. As a private practitioner I seldom see anyone who is properly balanced. This includes almost everyone from toddlers to ninety year olds. Virtually everyone needs to reestablish proper middle body muscle balance. The Rocking Chair Exercises promote middle body muscle balance.

2. Improve your diet. A healthy (heal-thy) diet can provide nutrients to your structures such as your knee and hip joints. This can help prevent structural pain problems with resultant weight gain.

A More Positive Frame Of Mind: The extra energy you get from Rocking Chair Exercises will usually result in a more positive frame of mind. This is partly because exercise causes your body to produce endorphins. Do you want a 'high' without drugs, alcohol, or tobacco? Try a daily dose of natural endorphins. Start having a daily routine of fresh foods, clean water, proper rest, exercise, and a positive mental attitude.

Agitated Or Nervous People: Rocking Chair Exercises may be of value in helping to calm agitated or nervous people. This includes the mentally challenged, by providing an outlet to help relieve their tension and hyperactivity. You may, after their middle body is physically conditioned for rocking at least five minutes, encourage them to rock for longer periods of time.

Physical Limitations Expanded: Another positive thing about Rocking Chair Exercises is that people with physical limitations, such as partly atrophied muscles may be able to work shoulder and rib muscles that often could not be used due to stress or injury. Aging joints and tense muscles should be moved several times a day. Rocking Chair Exercises provide easy movements that are controlled by the person who is exercising. They can adjust their activity to their level of tolerance and achievement. They don't have to worry about someone else controlling their movements and causing pain.

Physically Challenged: Rocking Chair Exercises may provide doable exercises to help some physically challenged people, to promote blood and lymph flow, strengthen their bodies, and promote relaxation.

Have Some Fun: You can make rocking chair exercising a social event and have some fun with family or friends. Whenever possible it's best to do your rocking chair exercising in the fresh air such as on a porch, patio, or screened-in area. This can be a great activity for young moms groups, bible studies, writing or reading clubs.

Results Of Rocking Chair Exercising: The following are results reported by patients who have tried the Rocking Chair Exercises:

*More energy.

*Feel better and calmer.

*Trimmer and stronger abs, obliques, hips, and thighs.

*Stronger low back with less of that 'rusty hinge' feeling.

*Promotes a smoothing of the skin around the abs, thighs, hips, and buns.

*Buns lifting up and becoming firmer.

*Women's breasts lifting up.

*Men's pectoral muscles moving up.

*Better appetite control.

*Raised metabolism.

*More strength in general.

*More stamina.

*Increased flexibility.

*Improved body balance.

*Better movement of the blood and lymph in major areas of the body.

*Flushing of toxins out of the body.

*Mood enhancement. Some mental health experts teach that it's difficult to worry and exercise at the same time. If you're really stressed, call a friend to rock with you until the feeling passes.

*An improved ability to walk or to engage in more demanding activities.

Chapter 9

Power Your Rock

One of the keys to getting maximum results with Rocking Chair Exercises is to provide your body with all of the elements it needs to rebuild and stretch. These include, but are not limited to, water and electrolytes.

Don't hydrate using just water. Exercise may use up a lot of electrolytes, such as calcium, sodium, and potassium, so it may be advisable to include an occasional sports drink to help replace the fluids and the electrolytes. Heavily sugared, high potassium, and artificially sweetened sports drinks are definitely not recommended. Caffeine is not recommended, as it's a diuretic, that is, it promotes kidney action to remove fluids out of the body. Caffeine is included in coffee, tea, colas, and many other drinks, including some root beers. One good idea is to simply add some fresh squeezed lemon juice to a water bottle. Apple juice and other fruit juices also work just as well.

Lifestyle And Nutrients: A healthy lifestyle and proper nutrition are essential parts of any exercise program. Exercise without proper nutrition is like having a flat tire on your vehicle. You pump up the tire and it looks okay, but then you just let it down without repairing the damage. You need to exercise to pump the nutrients into the various parts of the body including the joints. Even the best quality nutrients, such as water and glucosamine, will have trouble getting into the joints without exercise. Keep moving. Your heart pumps your blood but can be greatly assisted by

muscle action. What better muscle action is there than rocking chair exercising where the muscle action starts clear down at the feet?

Increase Fresh Food: Seek out fresh food sources. Good health comes primarily from good nutrition and the best sources of vitamins and minerals are found in fresh whole foods. Improving your nutrition would include drinking clean water, milk, and freshly squeezed juices; ingesting fresh healthy foods such as meat, fish, eggs, nuts, and figs, plus high-fiber multigrain breads and cereals, especially oatmeal (preferably the longer cooking type), raw vegetables, and water-rich fruits. My favorite fruits are apples (Ida Red variety), pears, plums, blueberries, blackberries, figs, dates, strawberries, and tomatoes. Tomatoes are served as a vegetable but botanically they're berries and therefore a fruit. Yogurt is usually a good food choice. For variety try buckwheat or whole- wheat pancakes instead of white flour pancakes. They don't have the same taste but they do have much different nutritional values. Foods from other lands and the seas are often a surprise taste and nutrition treat. Allergies to certain foods may limit your food choices.

People should seek foods and food supplements that are natural and prepared for market using exemplary quality control standards and manufacturing processes. It's also important to eat food that still has most or all of the food's life energy. Usually the more processed the food the lower the life energy. Fish and like foods should be from uncontaminated waters.

Calories: Cutting back on calories can be helpful but it is not as important as increasing physical activity to burn up extra weight. Many people who cut their

calories too low lose their energy and end up with health problems due to an inadequate intake of essential nutrients for health such as proteins, vitamins, minerals, and fats. If you incorporate a reduced calorie diet along with your exercise program, please always be careful to not go below the recommended calorie count for your height, weight, age, and activity level.

Fats: Cutting back on fats too much may result in major health consequences. Foods with fats are major sources of some important vitamins such as Vitamin A, which is needed for vision and other important body functions. Fats are also needed to protect vital organs such as the kidneys. Inadequate fat is suspect in some menstrual difficulties. Low levels of body fat may make estrogen levels drop too low to support reproductive system functions.

Synergism: Synergism is defined as "the mutually cooperating action of separate substances which together produce an effect greater than any component taken alone." I think of synergy as teamwork. I recall a story of several ranchers who conducted a test. They wanted to know how much weight a horse could pull. They harnessed up one horse to a wagon and the horse could pull 9,000 pounds. They figured that if one horse could pull 9,000 pounds then two horses harnessed together could pull 18,000 pounds. To their surprise the two horses harnessed together could pull 30,000 pounds. The synergy of the two horses working together was much greater than each horse working alone. Rocking Chair Exercises, along with good nutrition, is another example of synergy.

The synergy in fresh natural foods is remarkable. Low potencies of whole food synergistic vitamins are often much more effective than high potencies of fragmented vitamins. Isolating the nutrients often reduces their nutritional effect. The loss of the synergistic factors greatly reduces the synergetic results. The loss may also negate

some of the benefits attributed to a vitamin but which are actually the doings of one or more synergistic factors, which normally occur with the vitamin.

Chapter 10

Levels Of Exercises

Rocking Chair Exercises are broken into different levels. They are listed below:

1. Basic Rocking Chair Exercises: Everyone, young and old, should start at this level. This is designed for the beginner, the couch potato, the convalescent, and the world-class athlete. The Basic Exercises work virtually every important body part. The Basic Rocking Chair Exercises target the muscles of the feet, ankles, calves, shins, knees, inner and outer thighs, buns, hips, low back, abdomen, fingers, hands, wrists, forearms, elbows, shoulders, and upper and lower arms. The rocking action of the legs helps promote movement of the blood and lymph. The heart and lungs are mildly exercised and many important middle body muscles are activated.

2. Intermediate Rocking Chair Exercises: A well- rounded exercise program for people who wish to improve their muscle conditioning. Intermediate Rocking Chair Exercises, in addition to the same muscle areas as the Basic Rocking Chair Exercises, also target the waist, the obliques, and the neck, shoulder, chest, and upper back muscles.

3. Intense Rocking Chair Exercises: For the more dedicated exerciser. These are variations of the basic and intermediate exercises and are listed immediately after them. The Intense Rocking Chair Exercises target the same areas with the added benefit of more repetitions and changes in exercise angles of the neck, hands, arms,

and legs. The intense exercises challenge and strengthen the muscles and help build flexibility and stamina.

4. **Hand Strengthening: These are also variations and are listed immediately after other exercises. Hand strengthening exercises are included in the Rocking Chair Exercise program as having hand strength helps to deter arthritis in the hands, wrists, and elbows. The exercises help to provide power to handle normal everyday activities such as opening bottles of water. The hand strengthening exercises are very important for golfers and other people who need extra strength in their hands, wrists, and lower arms.**

5. **Rocking Chair Exercises Using Free Weights: This is a completely separate group of exercises that involve 1-5 pound weights. These exercises target the same areas as the Intermediate Rocking Chair Exercises but with resistance to strengthen the muscles and promote burning of fat deposits.**

6. **Rocking Chair Exercises Using Resistance Cords, Bands, or Tubing: This is a separate group of exercises that simulate bow and arrow motions. These exercises target the same areas as the Intermediate Rocking Chair exercises but with extra resistance from cords. This helps to strengthen the muscles and promote burning of fat deposits.**

7. **Rocking Chair Breathing Exercises: This group of exercises takes a little concentration. The breathing exercises gently work the respiration mechanisms. The lungs and bronchi are gently stimulated increasing the volume of air entering**

the body and helping to expel toxins from the body. Additionally, the breathing exercises work some of the internal core muscles. Breathing exercises, such as used in Lamaze training, have been found to help with pain and stress management.

8. Neck Imbalance Stretches: The neck has frequent problems with muscle weakness and/or imbalances. These stretches are needed by most people and will make many people feel better.

Start with the basic exercises, and then add exercises as you become stronger or feel that you are ready for them. You will get better results if you do these exercises on a daily basis. Exercise regularly to stay fit and move nutrients into your body cells.

Chapter 11

Positions Of Rocking Chair Exercises

Proper Sitting Position: Proper position, as in any exercise, is very important for the best results and for safety.

1. **Sit straight up with your low back against the back of the seat. Do not have any pads, such as a lumbar support, at the bottom of the back of the seat. Any pads or supports should extend evenly from the low back to the level of the top of the shoulders.**
2. **Place your shoeless feet firmly on the floor.**
3. **Rest your arms on the armrests. As an alternative, the most basic and relaxed arms position is with your hands hanging to the sides of the rocking chair. This will allow some elbow and shoulder joint movement with each rocking action. If there's no room next to the chair, place your hands, in a relaxed fashion, on your lap.**
4. **Relax your shoulders.**
5. **Do not lean your head backwards against the chair. You should exercise your neck muscles. There are many body functions that depend on having healthy neck muscles.**

Positions Of The Feet: Take off your shoes to allow more flexing of your ankles, arches, and toes. You may leave your socks on provided your socks aren't too tight or binding, thereby slowing blood circulation or restricting the flexing of your ankles, arches, and toes. Don't undermine the flexibility of your feet by wearing shoes all the time. You can become extremely clumsy when you lose that flexibility. Many people who have lost the flexibility of their ankles, arches, and toes end up on canes or walkers. Walk barefoot whenever you can, in foot-safe places, and do exercises, such as Rocking Chair Exercises, that flex your ankles, arches, and toes.

Orientation Of Body Parts: The orientation of various parts of the body is part of many of the Rocking Chair Exercises. The variations will place different stresses and stretches on different muscles such as the muscles of the arms, legs, and thighs. For example, a large muscle in the front side of each thigh, the quadriceps femoris, is considered to be one muscle. Some authorities classify the quadriceps as four muscles; the rectus femoris, vastus lateralis, vastus medialis, and vastus intermedius. These muscles are inserted by a common tendon below the knee area on the tuberosity of the tibia (shinbone). Each of the four muscle divisions has different origins on the pelvis, the greater trochanter (the boney projection on the top outside edge of the thigh), and the femur (thigh bone). Changing the orientation of the feet from duck-foot to pigeon-toed and back will work different parts of the quadriceps so you're getting more action out of each division of the muscle.

Each variation in exercise angle creates a different stress on different groups of muscles and tendons. This promotes flexibility and strength in the muscles and tendons helping to avoid those painful mini-strains from unaccustomed movements such as reaching or lifting.

Positions For Your Feet:

1. **Distance**: Varying the distance on how far your feet are in front of the Rocking Chair will determine whether your shin or calf muscles will get the greater workout.
2. **Spread**: There are three spread positions for your feet; close together, slightly spread apart, or spread far apart to the sides. The distance between your knees during Rocking Chair Exercises will determine which muscles, such as the inner or outer thigh muscles, will be worked the most.
3. **Orientation Of Your Feet**: The three feet orientation positions are:

A: Feet pointing straight ahead.

B: Duck-foot - having your toes pointing outward towards your sides like a duck.

C: Pigeon-toed - having your toes pointing inward towards each other like a pigeon.

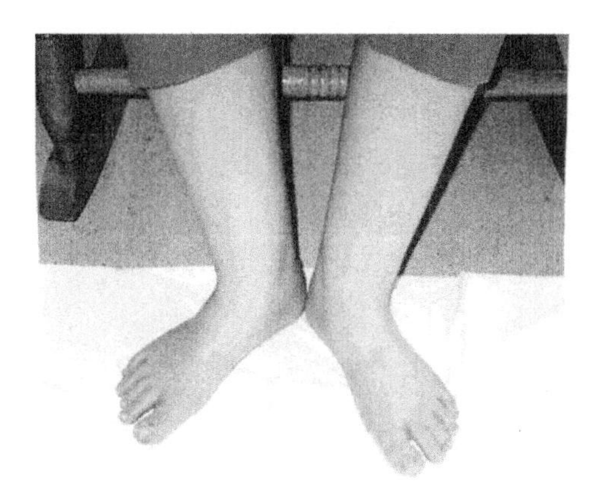

B: Duck-foot

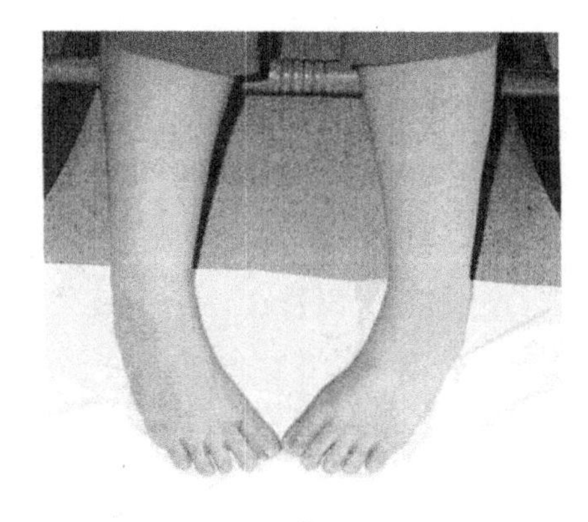

C: Pigeon-toed

Start with your feet, shoes off, in the duck-footed (toes turned outward) position. Rock one time, slightly raising your feet off the floor (or prop) and then turn your feet into the pigeon-toed (toes turned inward) position before your feet return to the floor. Change back and forth from the duck-footed to the pigeon-toed position with each rock. There are a few exercises, such as # 27 and 28, where your feet will not be touching the floor.

Positions Of The Toes And Ankles: There are two basic positions for your toes and ankles:

1. Having your toes pointed straight ahead.

2. Curling your toes and ankles upward.

Positions Of The Arms: Rest your arms on the armrests with your elbows against the back legs of the chair. Never lock your elbows during the exercises. Always keep your arms and elbows relaxed and flexible.

Positions Of The Hands: The first step is to mentally divide each armrest into three parts:

1. The front (distal or distant) 1/3rd portion.

2. The middle (medial) 1/3rd portion.

3. The back (proximal or close) 1/3rd portion.

Hand Positions: **There are four basic positions for the hands during hand exercises.**

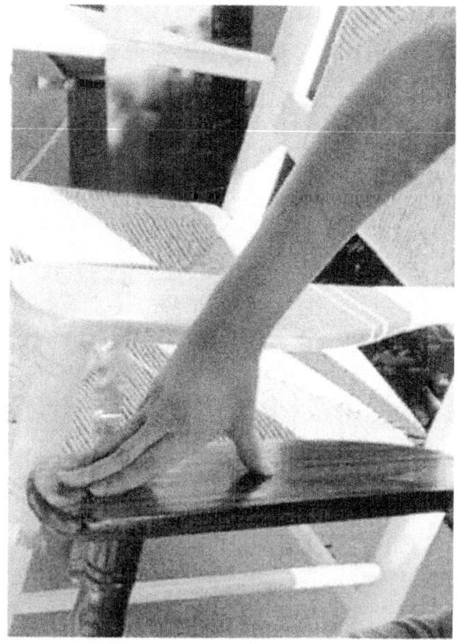
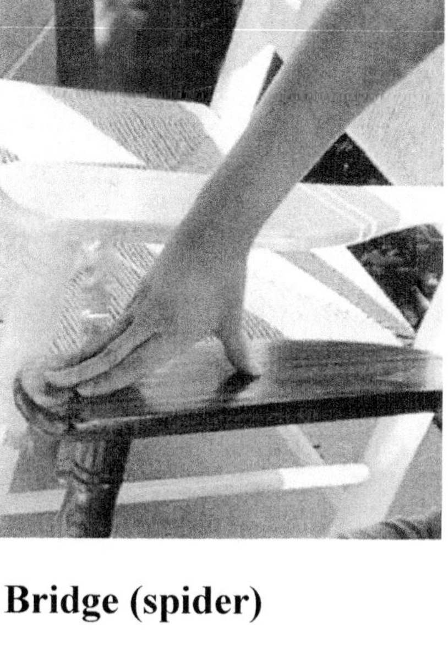

A: Bridge (spider)

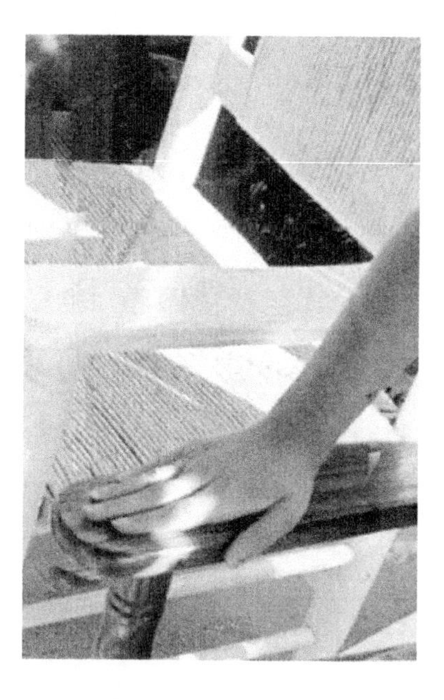

B: Flat handed

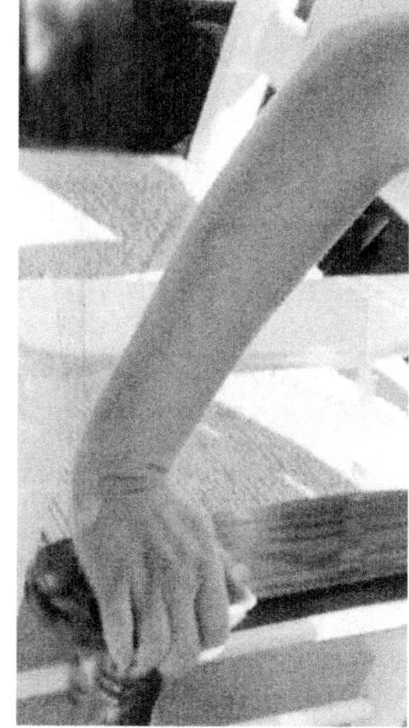

C: Wrapped inside

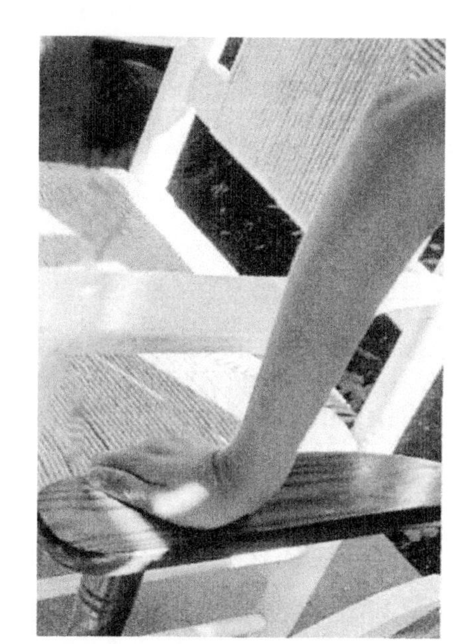

D: Wrapped outside

1. **Front (distal) 1/3rd Of Armrests:**

    1. **Bridge: Place your fingers on the front (distal) portions of the armrests, forming a bridge with your fingers, that is, placing your fingertips, spider fashion, on the front 1/3rd and then pressing down. Rock 4-10 times.**
    2. **Flat Handed: Place your fingers flat on the front 1/3rd of the armrests. Press down. Rock 4-10 times.**
    3. **Wrapped Inside: Wrap your hand onto or around the inside edge of the front 1/3rd of the armrests. Hold on and press down. Rock 4-10 times.**
    4. **Wrapped Outside: Wrap your hand onto or around the outside edge of the front 1/3rd of the armrest. Hold on and press down. Make sure you don't get your fingers jammed by nearby rocking chairs or other objects. Always protect your fingers. Depending on the shape of the armrests and the nearness of nearby objects you may not be able to wrap your fingers around the front 1/3rd but may be able to wrap around the medial or proximal parts of the armrests. Rock 4-10 times.**

2. **Middle (medial) 1/3rd Parts Of Armrests: Use the same hand and finger techniques as for the front (distal) 1/3rd of the armrests: bridge, flat handed, wrapped inside, and wrapped outside.**

3. **Back (proximal) 1/3rd Parts Of Armrests: Use the same hand and finger techniques as for the front (distal) and middle (medial) 1/3rds of the armrests: bridge, flat handed, wrapped inside, and wrapped outside.**

Do not substitute hand strengthening exercises, described later, for the above exercises. These exercises have different effects.

45s and 90s: There are 360 degrees in a circle. Imagine you're in the middle of the circle and you're facing the 0 (zero) degrees mark. Using Exercise # 21 Neck Exercises for an example, move your chin 45 degrees to the left side of your chest, letting your head hang toward the left side of your chest. Again, move your head another 45 degrees to your left side, so that your chin points toward your left shoulder. Stretch your neck by bringing your chin down toward your left shoulder. Then lean your head straight back so that you are looking at the ceiling or sky. Then move your head another 45 degrees so that your chin is pointing toward your right shoulder. Bring your chin toward your right shoulder. Continue another 45 degrees so that your chin is 45 degrees to the right of your chest, and drop your head so that it's hanging to the right side of your chest. Then bring your head back to center (0 degrees) and stretch your neck by moving your chin to your chest. You will have then rotated your head 360 degrees and stretched your neck muscles effectively but gently.

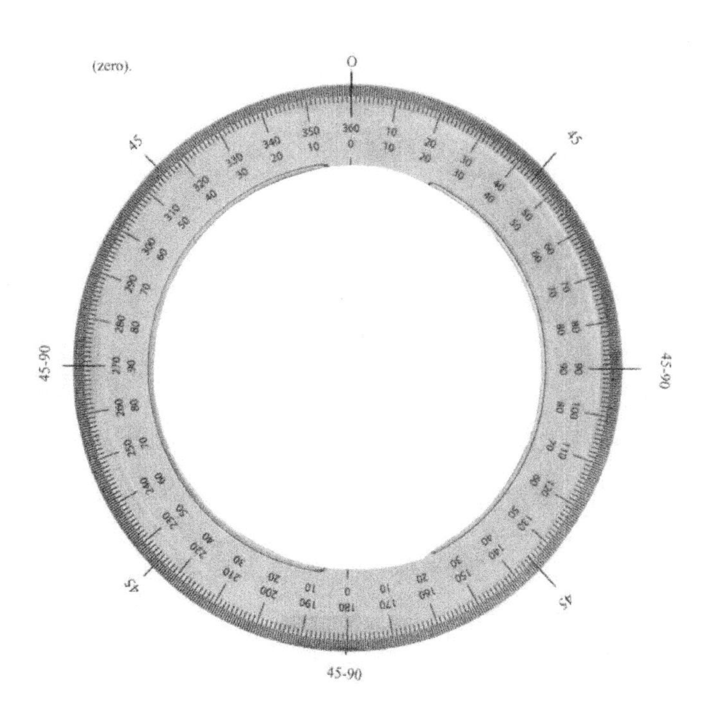

45s: This relates to moving a body part 45 degrees in some direction. For example, during Neck 45s Exercise (# 21c), you're moving your chin 45 degrees so that your chin is pointing over the right side of your chest. Then move your chin another 45 degrees so that your chin is pointing towards your left shoulder. These aren't necessarily perfect 45-degree moves; we're using approximate degrees. In some cases, a person may not be able to move into a position because it's constrained by being too close to an object or the person may not have the flexibility to actually achieve that 45-degree change. Just do what's comfortable for you.

90s: This relates to moving a body part 90 degrees in some direction. For example, during the Arm Circles Exercises (# 19) Intense, your thumbs are turned from facing downward to facing forward. This isn't necessarily a perfect 90- degree move but we're using approximate degrees. In some cases, a person may not be able to move into a position because it's constrained by being too close to an object or the person not having the flexibility to actually achieve that 90-degree change. Just do what's comfortable for you.

45s and 90s: Some exercises will involve both 45s and 90s.

Axilla (Armpit) Stretches: (Exercise # 7) Axilla Stretches should be an important part of any exercise session. The muscles in this area are either cooperating with and/or affecting a lot of external and internal muscles such as the muscles around the heart, bronchial tubes, and lungs.

Foot Wags: (Exercise # 14) Extend your left leg directly forward and sway your foot from side-to-side like a dog wagging its tail. Rock 4-10 times. Return your

left foot to the floor. Then wag your right foot. This exercise challenges the knees, hamstrings, and the inner and outer thighs. This may be a rather clumsy move but it'll become smoother with time. Wag only one foot at a time to prevent exerting too much swayback stress into the low back curve.

Neck Exercises: (Exercise 21) The Neck Exercises help to stretch out the neck muscles and also tone the jowls, the fleshy part of the lower jaw.

Triceps Stretches: (Exercises # 24, 25 and 35) Helps prevent minor pulled muscle problems due to reaching backwards such as retrieving something from the back seat of a car while the person is sitting in the front seat.

Knees Up And In: (Exercise # 28) Number 28 may not be possible for some people so don't hurt yourself trying too hard. Do what's comfortable for you. For some people, it's best to forget this exercise for a long time until they get enough flexibility. Some people who are totally limber may not understand limitations of flexibility since it's so easy for them. For example, a young woman took her 10yearold daughter to her yoga class. Some of the yoga exercises that were torturous for the mother were a breeze for her flexible young daughter.

Steering Wheel: (Exercise # 40) Imagine you're driving through the mountains and there are a lot of hairpin curves, some curving to the left and every other turn curving right.

a. Hold one weight (steering wheel) in both hands and directly in front of

you. Similar to turning the steering wheel on an automobile, make a hard left and then a hard right.

b. Alternate steering back and forth while rocking.

This creates a very active workout for the abdominal, arm, shoulder, rib cage, and upper and middle back muscles including the trapezius and erector spinae muscles. These muscles were used a lot in the old days before power steering was introduced.

<u>Neck Muscles Imbalance</u>: (Exercise # 49) Many people have severe problems with neck muscle imbalances. The average person doing neck exercises sits or stands straight up and then nods their neck 'yes' (pecks) and then 'no' and then rolls their head from side-to-side. The problem with this process is that the weight of the head, like the weight of a bowling ball, crunches down on the muscle fibers and causes them to compress. The function of muscles is to contract and you don't want the neck muscles to either contract or compress when you want to release muscle tension. The neck muscles really don't stretch well when you do exercises that use the head as a bowling ball pushing down on the muscle fibers from above. You want to release the muscle tension and not increase the tension in the neck muscles. You want to stretch the muscle fibers.

I ask my patients to do the yes, no, and neck rolls exercises but while reversing gravity. The patient is to lie on their stomach on a bed and let their head hang over the edge of the bed like they're heaving (throwing up). Their head must be kept lower than their neck thereby using the weight of their head, like a bowling ball, to help stretch the muscle fibers. The patient is instructed not to try to work the neck muscles hard, as this will cause contractions of the muscles instead of releasing the

muscle tension. They're to think of their head as a ball on a string and act like a kitten is softly pushing their head from side-to-side and back and forth.

An alternative to this is to lean over while holding onto a chair or other surface for stability. Be careful to hold onto something in case you get dizzy. Then do the same exercises, keeping your head lower than your neck. You should hang your head directly between your elbows. You really get a good muscle stretch using your head as a weight and allowing a free-flowing movement of the neck muscles. This promotes the release of neck muscle tension and better neck muscle balance.

Chapter 12

Basic Rocking Chair Exercises

<u>Precautions</u>: The precautions from Chapter 3 are repeated below, as many people tend to skip the narrative in the front of exercise books and go right to the exercises. A full explanation, the whys and why-nots, of the precautions are given in Chapter 3.

1. **See your Doctor before starting any diet or exercise program.**
2. **Do not eat and then do Rocking Chair Exercises. Wait at least one hour after eating before doing Rocking Chair Exercises.**
3. **Fit the rocking chair to your body size.**
4. **Do not sit forward on the front edge of the seat.**
5. **Do not keep both of your legs outstretched in front of you while rocking.**
6. **Do not use a lumbar support.**
7. **Do only a few repetitions of each exercise.**
8. **Remove keys, wallets, etc. from your back pockets.**

Basic Rocking Chair Exercises:

#1. Sit And Rock

A. **Remove your shoes and place your feet flat on the floor with your toes in the duck-footed (toes pointing outward) position.**

B. **Sit straight up with your back against the back of the chair. Your upper and lower back should be close to or touching the back of the chair.**

C. **Hold on to the front edge of the armrests. As an alternative, you may choose to let your arms and hands hang to the sides of the rocking chair. If there's no room next to the chair, place your hands, in a relaxed fashion, on your lap.**

D. **Your knees should be a comfortable 3 to 12 inches apart.**

E. **Relax your shoulders. Relax - let go of the tension. Rock easily backwards and then let the rocking chair rebound forward on its own. Your rhythm may be clumsy at first but should smooth out after a while.**

F. **With the first rock, change the position of your feet from duck-footed (toes pointing outward) to pigeon-toed (toes pointing inward, toward each**

other). Then alternate between duck-footed and pigeon-toed on each rock. Alternating the position of your feet will work the muscles of your ankles, knees, inner and outer thighs, hips, and buns.

G. At first, limit your rocking time to 5 minutes or 150 rocks. Rocking too long at first may result in muscle cramps and/or bruising of the skin. You may want to rest a while and then resume rocking. After your middle body (core) conditioning improves you can rock to your heart's content or until your middle body muscles tighten up and refuse to rock any more.

2 Finger Exercises

Keep moving your feet and alternating from duck-footed to pigeon-toed and back.

A. Place your fingers, both hands at the same time, in a bridge or spider fashion, on the front (distal) 1/3rd of the armrests. This position is shown in chapter 11. Push down with your finger- tips. Rock 4-10 times.
B. Flatten your hands onto the front part of the armrests. Push down on the armrests to increase resistance. Rock 4-10 times.
C. Turn your hands so that your fingers are facing inwards. Grasp the front inside of the armrests and push down to increase resistance. Rock 4-10 times.
D. Turn your hands so that your fingers are facing outwards. Avoid objects that may jam your fingers. Grasp the front outside of the armrests and push down to increase resistance. Rock 4-10 times.

E. Move your hands back to the middle 1/3rd third of the armrests.
Repeat the finger movements: bridge, flat, inside, and then outside.
Rock 4-10 times.

F. Move your hands to the back (proximal) 1/3rd of the armrests.
Repeat the finger movements: bridge, flat, inside, and then outside.
Rock 4-10 times.

3 Hand Strengthening (football squeeze)

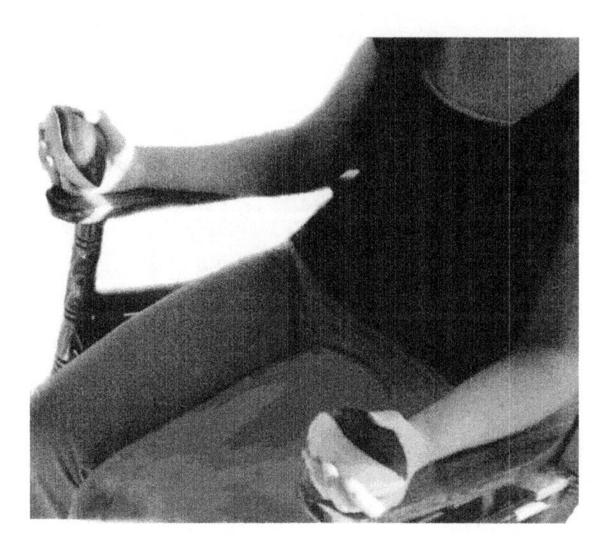

Hold your arms just above the armrests. Holding a mini sponge football in each hand, squeeze the footballs each time you rock backwards. Relax your grip as the rocking chair rebounds.

Rock 4-10 times.

Intense: Do the 90s with the footballs as you squeeze and release, thumbs down, thumbs inward, upward and then outward.

(Rotate your hands 90 degrees)

The 90s are explained in more detail on page 61.

4 Hands-Behind-Head

Lace your fingers behind your head and stay in that position.

A: Crunches:

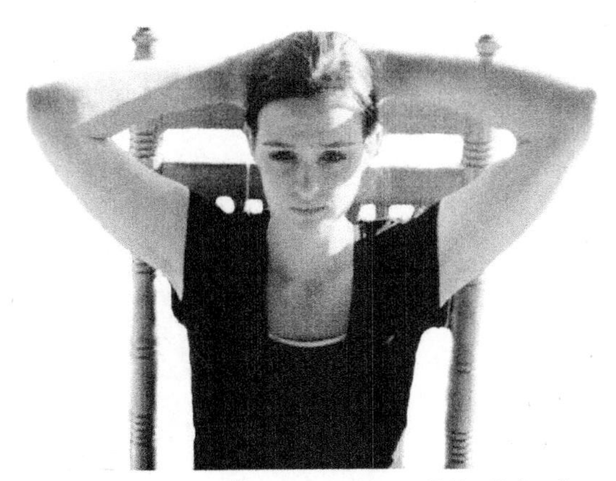

Sit straight up, with your fingers laced behind your head.

Rock 4-10 times.

B: Side Crunches:

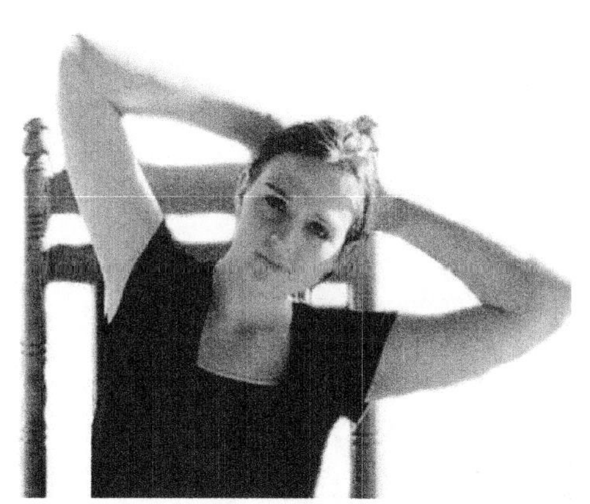

Stay in that upright position and bend over toward your left side.

Remain in that bent over position. Rock 4-10 times.

Reverse - bend to your right side. Rock 4-10 times.

B: Side Crunches:

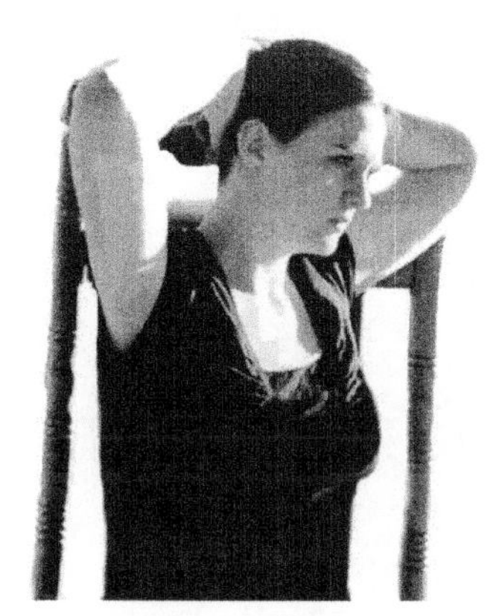

Stay in the hands-behind-head position and twist to your left as far as you can. Your left elbow should be pointing towards the left finial, which is behind you. Stay in that position and rock 4-10 times. Reverse - twist towards the right finial as far as you can. Rock 4-10 times.

D: Tilt Side-To-Side:

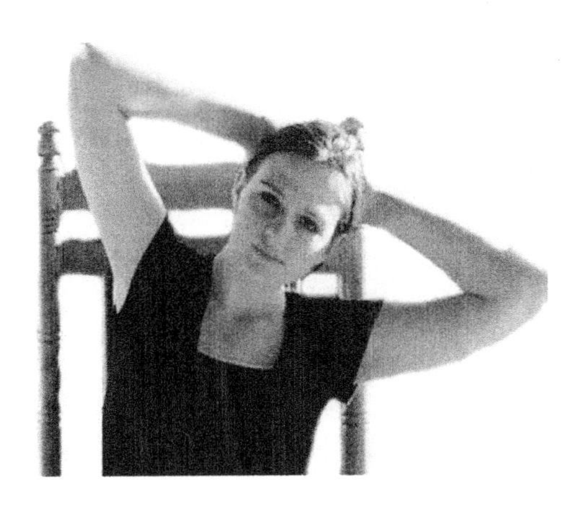

Tilt alternately from side-to-side.

Rock 4-10 times.

E: Oblique Crunches:

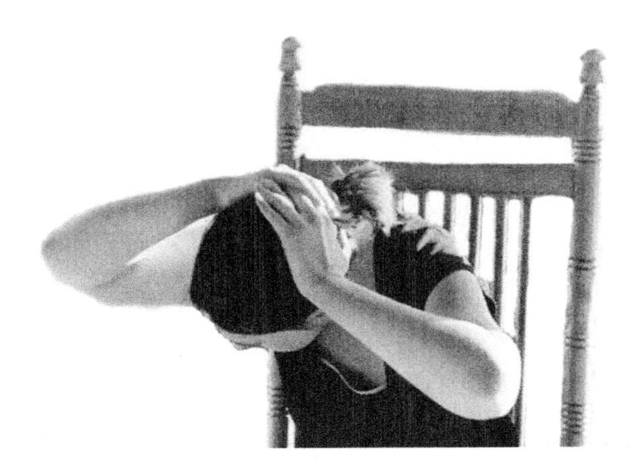

Keep your hands laced behind your head and twist forward pointing your left elbow towards the front of the right armrest.

Twist as far as is comfortable - do not overstretch.

Straighten up and twist forward pointing your right elbow towards the left armrest. Alternate crunching to your right and then to your left. Rock 4-10 times.

Chapter 13

Intermediate Rocking Chair Exercises

5 Rib Stretches

Keep moving your feet, as with almost all Rocking Chair Exercises, alternating from duck-footed to pigeon-toed and back.

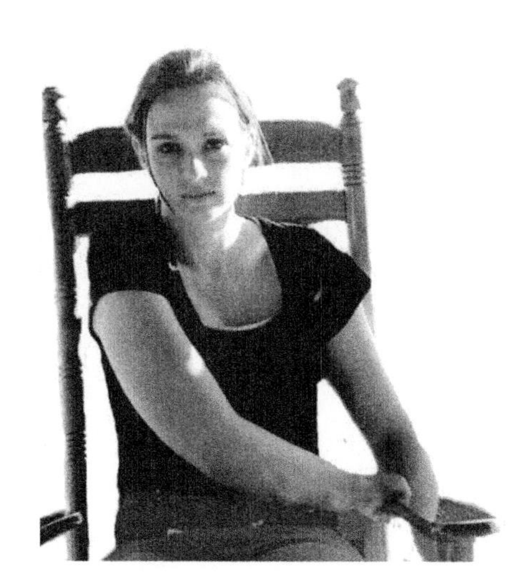

A. **Relax your left arm and let it hang to the side of the chair. Cross your right hand over the middle of your body and grasp the back (proximal) 1/3rd of the left armrest. Rock 4-10 times.**
B. **Relax your right arm and let it hang to the side of the chair. Using your left hand, grasp the back 1/3rd of the right armrest. Rock 4-10 times.**
C. **Cross your hands, your right hand on the left armrest and the left hand on the right armrest. Grasp the middle 1/3rd or whatever you can reach of both armrests. Rock 4-10 times.**

6 Pectoral Muscle Stretches

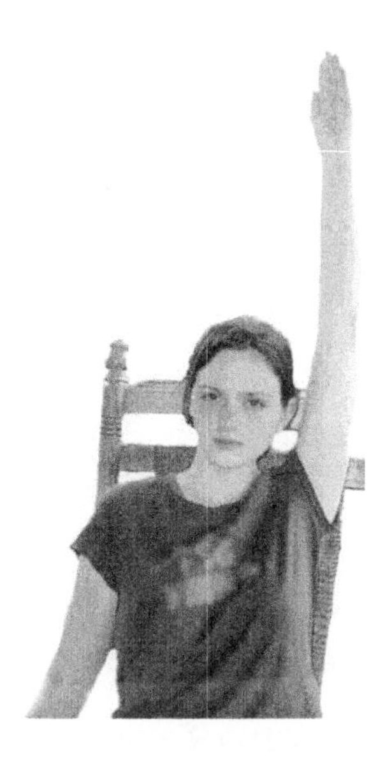

A. **Left Pectoral Stretch:** Let your right arm and hand hang to the side of the chair. Extend your left arm straight up and a little towards behind your back as far as is comfortable. Rock 4-10 times.

B. **Right Pectoral Stretch:** Let your left arm and hand hang to the side of the chair. Extend your right arm straight up and a little towards behind your back as far as is comfortable. Rock 4-10 times.

Intense: Turn your hands, left hand first, in a 90s action. Twist your hands so that your thumbs are pointing forward, then inward, then backward, then outward.

Hand Strengthening: Holding a mini football in each hand, squeeze each time you rock backwards and relax your grip as the rocking chair rebounds.

7 Axilla (armpit) Stretches

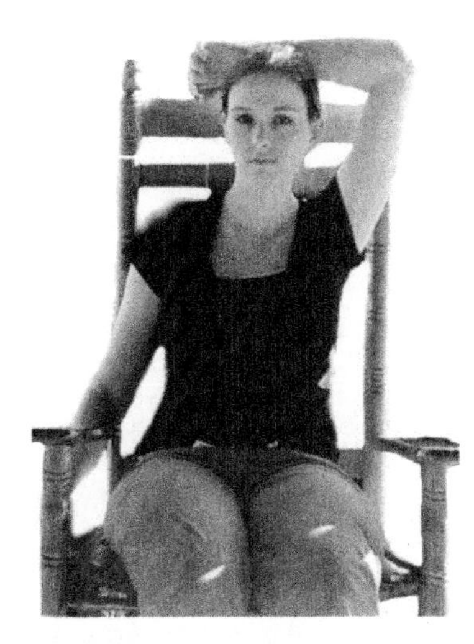

A. **Left Elbow Bent Behind Head:** Let your right arm and hand hang to the side of the chair. Raise your left arm, bent at the elbow, and let your left arm relax just behind the top of your head. Rock 4-10 times.

B. **Right Elbow Bent Behind Head:** Let your left arm and hand hang to the side of the chair. Raise your right arm, bent at the elbow, and let your right arm relax just behind the top of your head. Rock 4-10 times.

Hand Strengthening: **Holding a mini football in each hand, squeeze each time you rock backwards and relax your grip as the rocking chair rebounds.**

8 Arms To The Sky

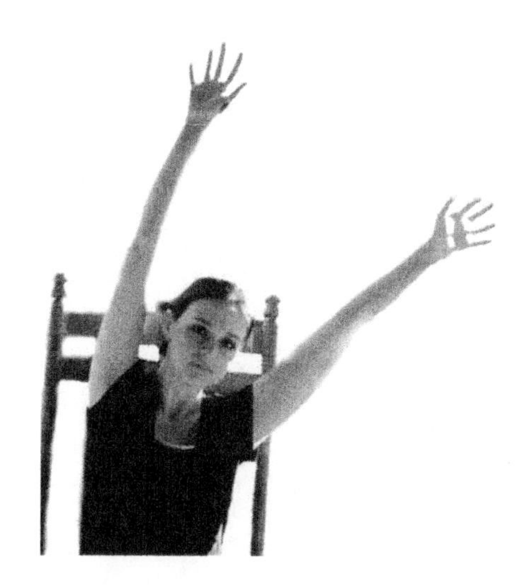

A. Raise both arms directly over your head. Rock 4-10 times.

B. While keeping your arms up, lean over to your left side as far as possible and stay in that leaning position as you rock.
Rock 4-10 times.

C. Reverse - lean over to your right side. Rock 4-10 times.

Hand Strengthening: Holding a mini football in each hand, Squeeze the football each time you rock backwards and relax your grip as the rocking chair rebounds.

9 Arms Up And Twist

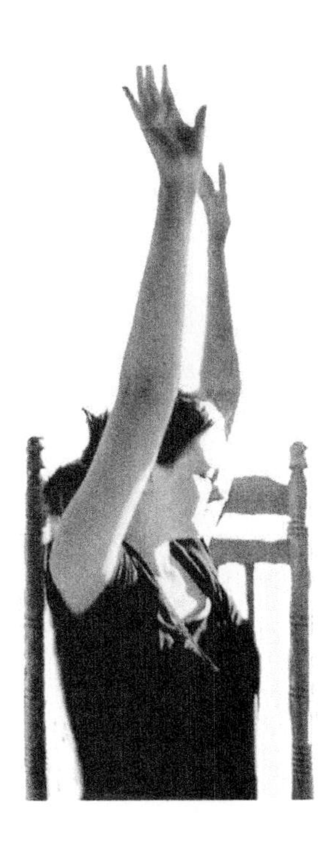

A. **Twist Left**: Keep your arms up and twist your body toward the left finial as far as possible. Rock 4-10 times.

B. **Twist Right**: Keep your arms up and twist your body toward the right finial as far as possible. Rock 4-10 times.

Hand Strengthening: Holding a mini football in each hand, squeeze each time you rock backwards and relax your grip as the rocking chair rebounds.

 # 10 Tilt Side-To-Side

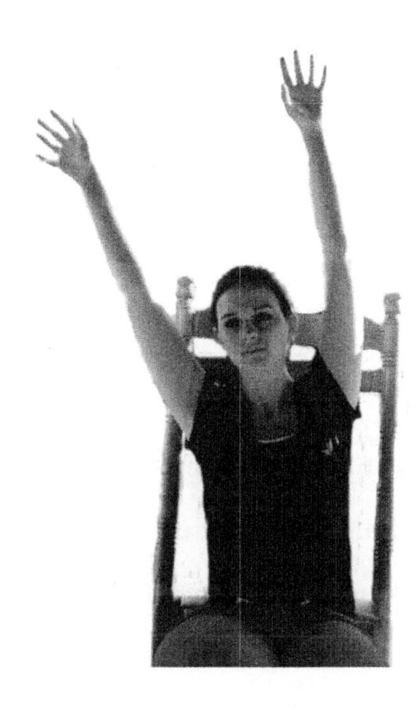

A. **Tilt To The Right: Keep your hands up and tilt to the right.**
   Rock 4-10 times.

B. **Tilt To The Left: Keep your hands up and tilt to the left.**
   Rock 4-10 times.

Hand Strengthening: Holding a mini football in each hand, squeeze each time you rock backwards and relax your grip as the rocking chair rebounds.

11 Hand Crossovers

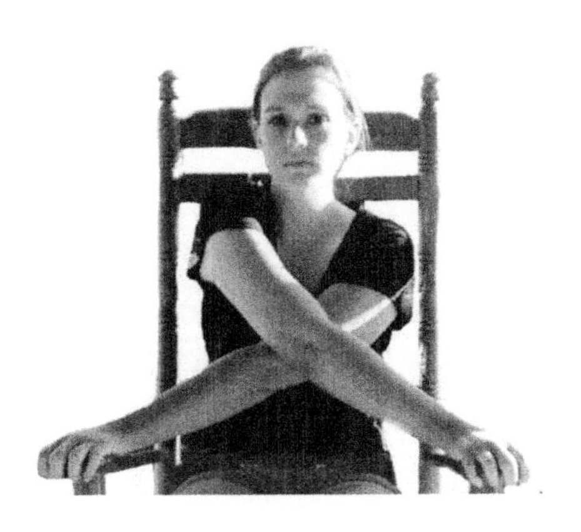

A. **Right- Hand Crossover:**

Place your left hand on the front of the right armrest and your right hand on the front of the left armrest. Your right elbow should be above your left elbow. Lean backwards until you feel a stretching sensation in the muscles along the ribs in your upper back area.

Rock 4-10 times.

B. **Left Hand Crossover: Reverse - Use the same hand positions But your left elbow should be above your right elbow.**

Rock 4-10 times.

12 Trapezius Muscles Stretches

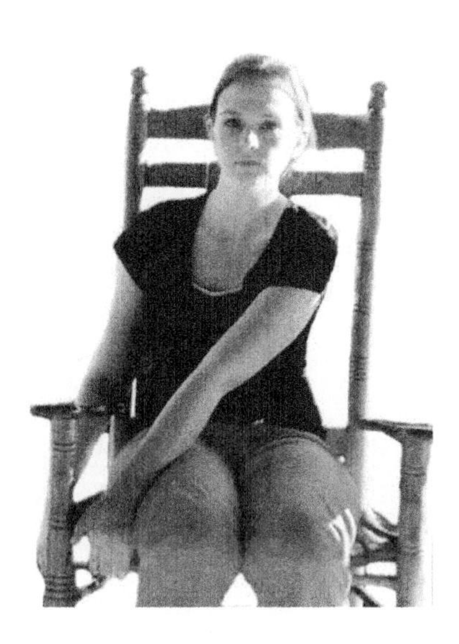

A. **Left Trapezius Stretch: Let your right arm hang to the side of the right armrest. Using your left hand, reach across and grasp the front of the seat just to the side of your right knee. Hold on and rock 4-10 times.**

B. **Right Trapezius Stretch: Reverse - Let your left arm hang to the side of the left armrest. Using your right hand, reach across and grasp the front side of the seat just to the side of your left knee. Rock 4-10 times.**

C. **Trapezius Muscles Stretch**: Using both hands, grasp the center of the front of the seat between your knees and hold on firmly. Let your head hang forward. Rock 4-10 times.

13 Knee Kicks

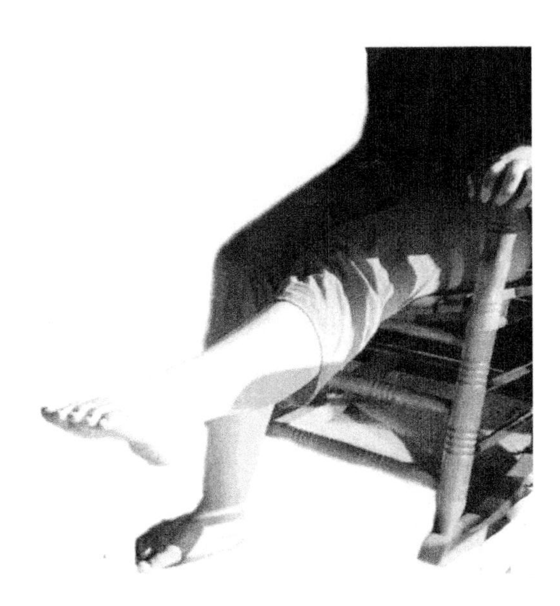

A. Swing your left foot forward and up. Point your toes straight ahead and rock backwards. Curl your ankles, arches, and toes up and backwards as you return your foot to the floor position.

B. Reverse - use your right foot.

Intense: While rocking, move your feet, left foot first, in a 90s action so that your toes point inward, then straight ahead, and finally outward.

Hand Strengthening: Holding a mini football in each hand, squeeze each time you rock backwards and relax your grip as the rocking chair rebounds.

14 Foot Wags (thighs abduction and adduction)

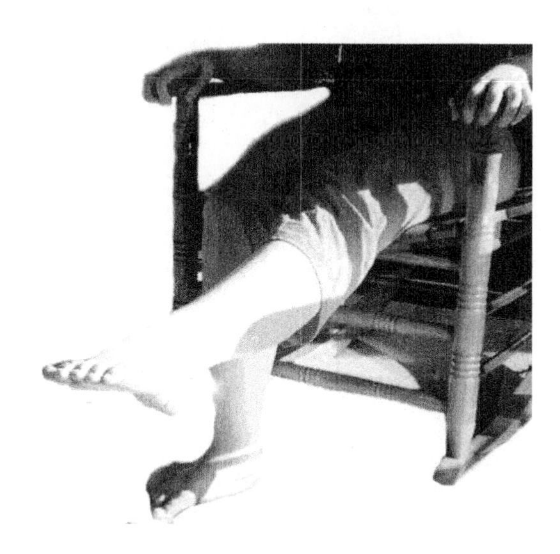

A. Hold your left leg straight out in front of you. Wag your left foot from side-to side as you rock. Rock 4-10 times.

B. Hold your right leg straight out in front of you. Wag your right foot from side-to-side as you rock. Rock 4-10 times.

Intense: While rocking, move your feet, left foot first, in a 90s action: toes inward toward each other, toes straight ahead, then toes outward.

Hand Strengthening: Holding a mini football in each hand, squeeze each time you rock backwards and relax your grip as the rocking chair rebounds.

15 Knee Lifts To Opposite Side

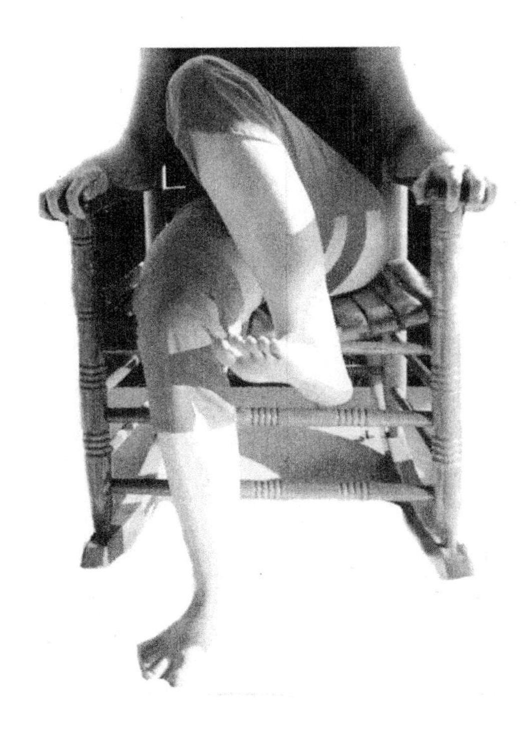

A. Pull your left knee up toward the right side of your chest as you rock backwards. Point your toes straight ahead when lifting your knee. Curl your ankles, arches and toes up as you rebound, and then return your foot to the floor. Rock 4-10 times.

B: Pull your right knee up toward the left side of your chest as you rock backwards. Point your toes straight ahead when lifting your knee. Curl your ankles, arches and toes up as you rebound, and then return your foot to the floor. Rock 4-10 times.

<u>**# 16 Ankle And Calf Stretches**</u>

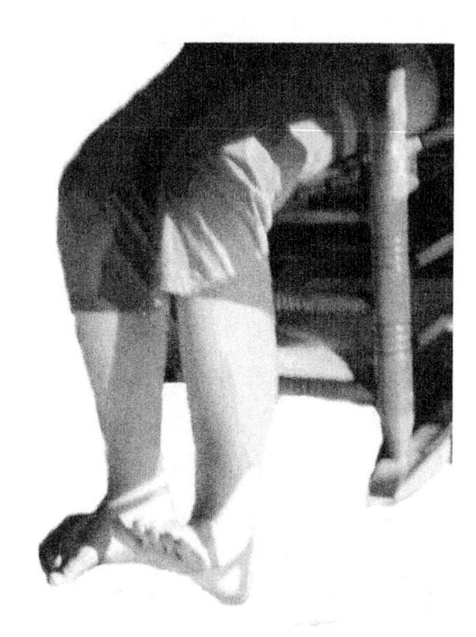

Do not exercise both legs at the same time as it may stress the muscles of the lower back curve.

A. **Raise your left foot slightly above the floor. Point your toes straight ahead and rock backwards. Curl your ankles, arches, and toes on the rebound motions. Rock 4-10 times.**
B. **Reverse - Raise your right foot slightly above the floor. Point your toes straight ahead and rock backwards. Curl your ankles, arches, and toes on the rebound motions. Rock 4-10 times.**

<u>Intense</u>: While rocking, move your feet, left foot first, in a 90s action. Toes inward toward each other, then toes straight ahead, and finally toes outward.

Hand Strengthening: Holding a mini football in each hand, squeeze each time you rock backwards and relax your grip as the rocking chair rebounds.

17 Angel Stretch 45s To The Sky

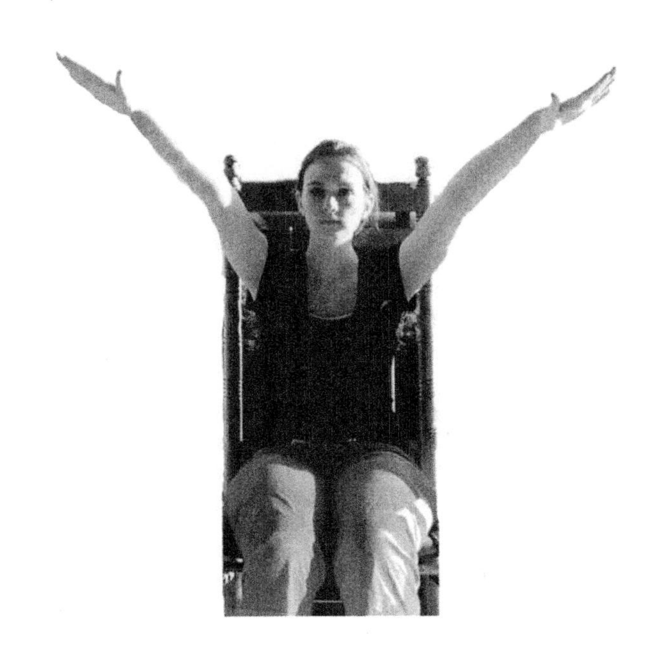

A. Hold your arms straight out in front of you, reaching for the sky at about a 45-degree angle and with your palms facing down. Rock 4-10 times.
B. Move your arms 45 degrees towards your sides while keeping your arms up at a 45-degree angle. Rock 4-10 times.
C. Hold your arms directly out to your sides and up at a 45-degree angle. Rock 4-10 times.

Intense: While stretching your arms upward, rotate your hands in a 90 action.

Hand Strengthening: Holding a mini football in each hand, squeeze each time you rock backwards and relax your grip as the rocking chair rebounds.

18 Arm Stretches 45s

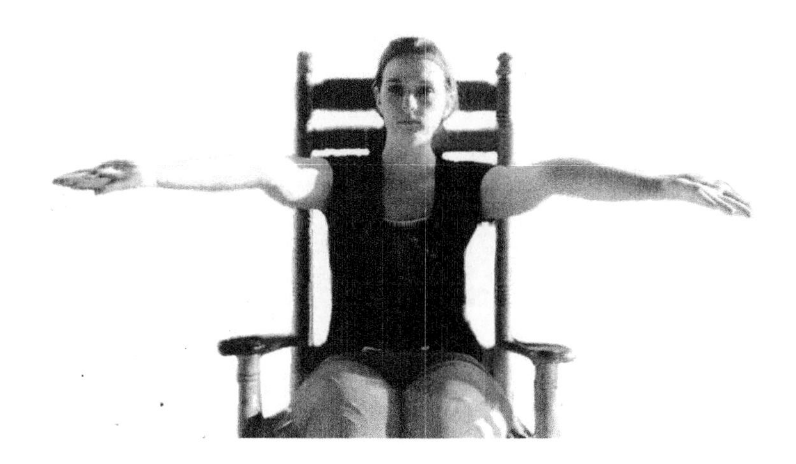

A. **Hold your arms straight out in front of you, chest high, and with your palms facing up. Rock 4-10 times.**
B. **Hold your arms out, chest high, at a 45-degree angle. Rock 4-10 times.**
C. **Hold your arms straight out to your sides, chest high. Rock 4-10 times.**

Intense: While stretching, rotate both hands in a 90s action.

Hand Strengthening: Holding a mini football in each hand, squeeze each time you rock backwards and relax your grip as the rocking chair rebounds.

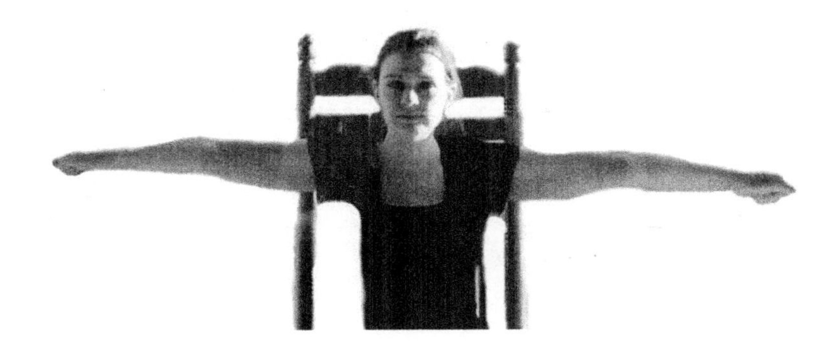

A. <u>Arms Circling Forward</u>: **Extend your hands out directly to your sides. Relax your shoulders. Rotate your arms forward and then all the way around in a circular motion. Rock 4-10 times.**

B. <u>Arms Circling Backward</u>: **Reverse - rotate your arms backwards and then all the way around in a circular motion. Rock 4-10 times.**

<u>Intense</u>: While circling with your arms, rotate both hands in a 90s action. Thumbs downward, thumbs forward, thumbs upward and then thumbs backwards.

<u>Hand Strengthening</u>: Holding a mini football in each hand, squeeze each time you rock backwards, and relax your grip as the rocking chair rebounds.

20 Shoulder Shrugs

Relax your shoulders. Tense shoulders don't move easily.

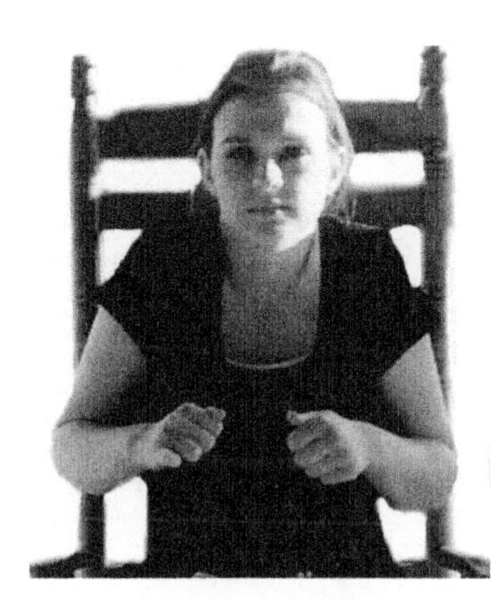

A. **Shoulders Shrugging Forwards: Lift and rotate your shoulders upwards and forward in a cycling motion. Rock 4-10 times.**

B. **Shoulders Shrugging Backwards: Reverse – lift and rotate your shoulders upwards and backwards in a cycling motion. Rock 4-10 times.**

Intense: While shrugging, rotate both hands in a 90s action. Thumbs inward, thumbs up, and then thumbs outward.

Hand Strengthening: Holding a mini football in each hand, squeeze each time you rock backwards and relax your grip as the rocking chair rebounds.

21 Neck 45s

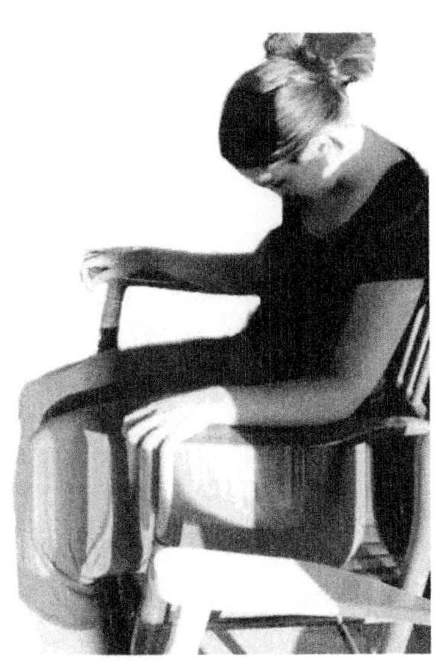

A. **Sit erect and let your head hang towards the center of your chest. Place your hands on the armrests or let your hands hang to your sides. Relax your shoulders. Rock 4-10 times.**

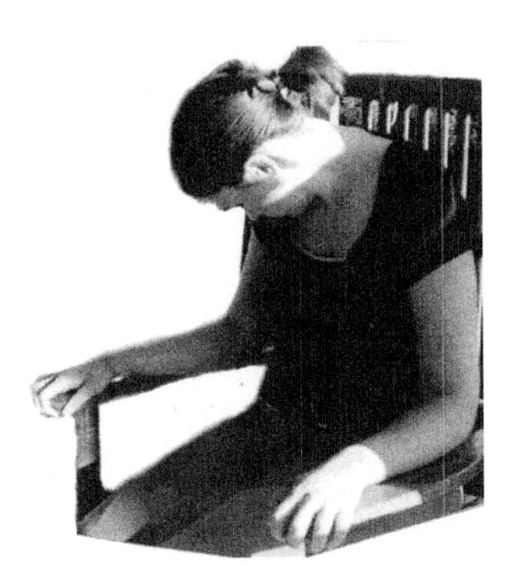

B. **Move your chin 45 degrees to the right side of your chest, letting Your head hang towards the right side of your chest. Rock 4-10 times.**

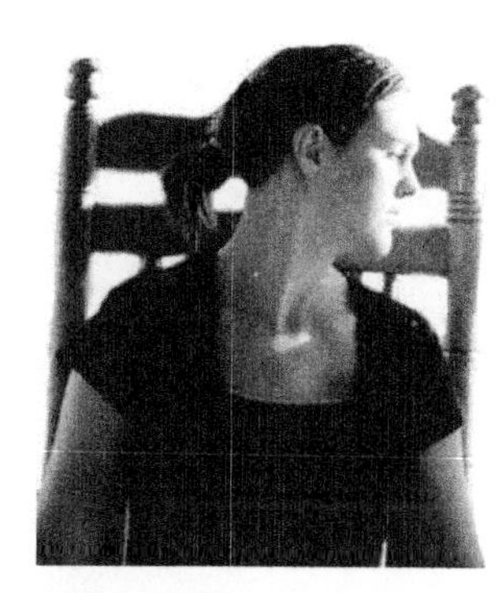

C. Move your chin another 45 degrees to your right so that your chin points toward your right shoulder. Rock 4-10 times.

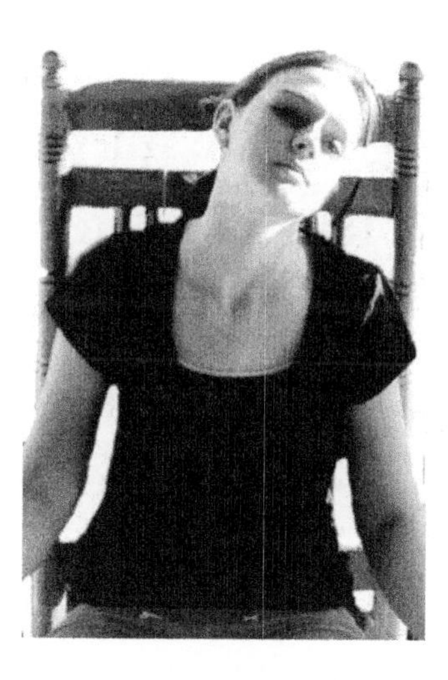

D. Move your head another 45 degrees, letting your head hang backwards toward the right final. Rock 4-10 times.

E. Sit erect and tilt your head backwards toward the middle of the back of the chair. Don't lean your head against the chair. Rock 4-10 times.

F. Move your head 45 degrees toward the left finial, letting your head hang backwards toward the finial. Rock 4-10 times.

G. **Move your chin 45 degrees to your left so that your chin points toward your left shoulder. Rock 4-10 times.**

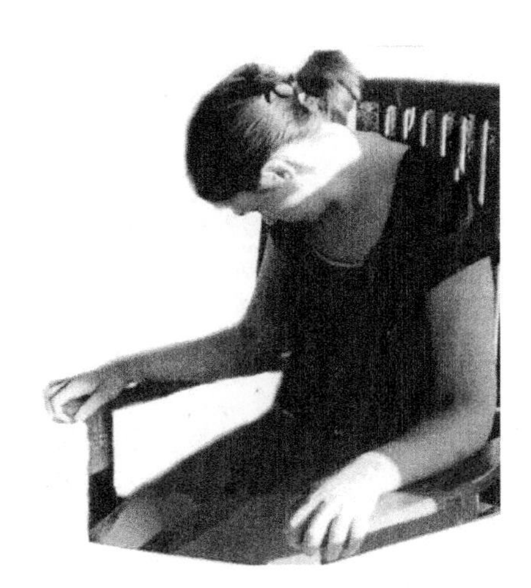

H. **Move your chin 45 degrees forward, letting your head hang towards the left side of your chest. Rock 4-10 times.**

I. **Return to the starting point. Let your chin hang forwards toward the center of your chest. Rock 4-10 times.**

Intense: 45s and 90s. In each 45-degree position, rotate your head, in a 90-degree fashion, first to the left, then to the right, and then to the middle.

 # 22 Ear Pull

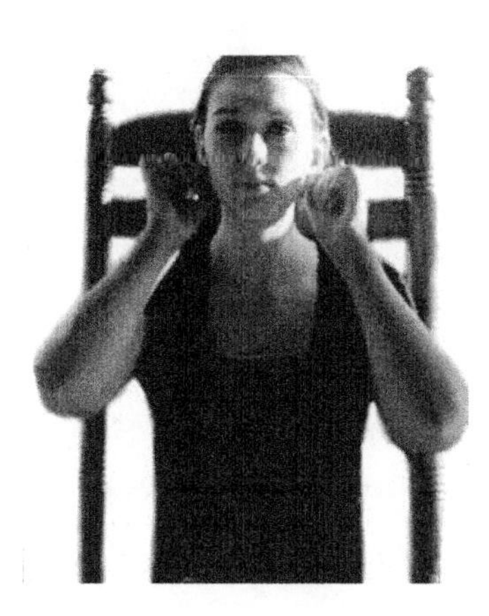

A. **Ear Lobes: Using both hands, grasp the bottoms of your ears (earlobes). Hold your earlobes lightly while exerting a soft downward and outward pulling stretch on your earlobes. Do not pull hard.**

Rock 4-10 times.

B. **Ear Crest: Using both hands, lightly hold the tops of your ears (crests). Hold your ears softly while exerting a soft upward and outward pull on your ear crests. Do not pull hard.**

Rock 4-10 times.

23 Biceps Stretch

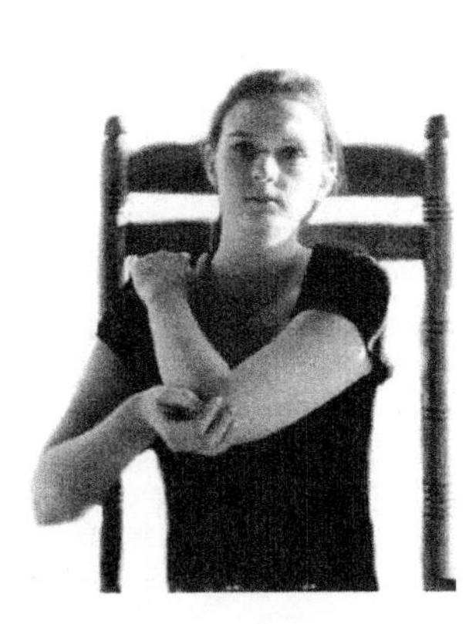

A. **Cross your left arm across your chest, keeping your elbow bent and touching your chest (sternum area). The fingers of your left hand should be relaxed and resting on your right shoulder. Using your right hand, grasp your left elbow and pull your left elbow gently and directly towards your right side. This will give a good stretch to your left biceps. Rock 4-10 times.**

B. **(Reverse): Cross your right arm across your chest, keeping your elbow bent and touching your chest. Using your left hand, pull your right elbow gently and directly towards your left side. Rock 4-10 times.**

 # 24 Triceps Stretch

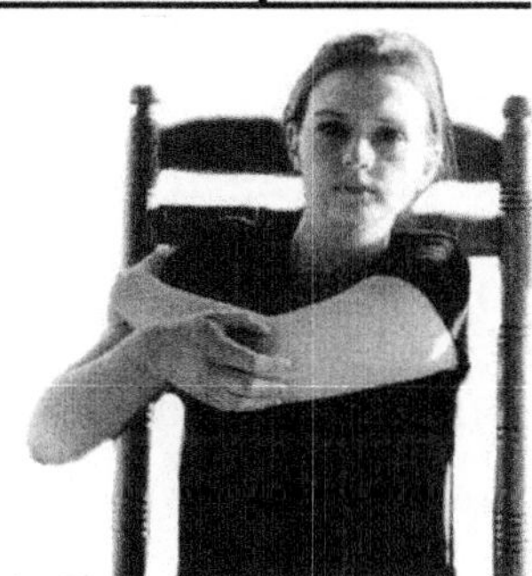

A. **Using your left arm, reach straight across your chest with your elbow in the air in front of you. With your right hand, reach and grasp your left elbow.**
   Pull your left elbow directly towards your right side as you rock.
   Rock 4-10 times.

B. **Using your right arm, reach straight across your chest with your elbow in the air in front of you. With your left hand, reach and grasp your right elbow.**
   Pull your right elbow towards your left side as you rock.
   Rock 4-10 times.

25 Triceps Overhead Stretch

A. Raise your left arm and hold it slightly behind your head. Bend your arm at the elbow. Reach over your head with your right hand and grasp your left elbow. Pull it gently towards your right side as you rock.
   Rock 4-10 times.

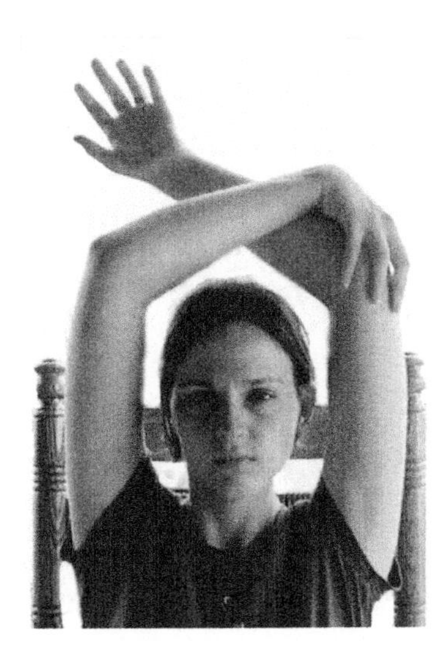

B. Raise your right arm and hold it slightly behind your head. Bend your arm at the elbow. Reach over your head with your left hand and grasp your right elbow. Pull it gently towards your left side as you rock.
   Rock 4-10 times.

26 Wrist Stretches

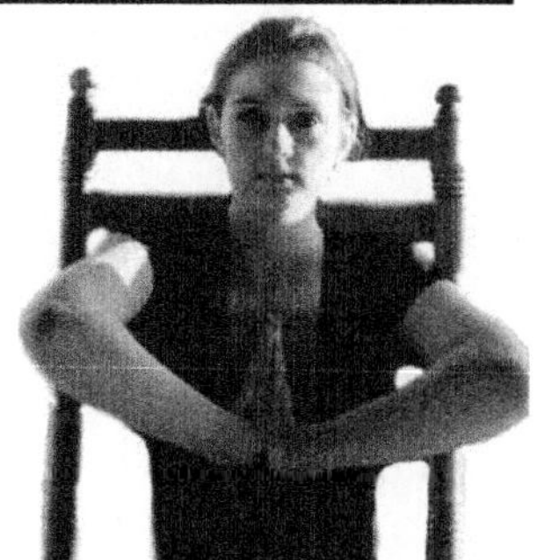

A. Hold your hands together and tight against the front of your chest (sternum). Your fingers should be pointing straight up similar to a praying position. Keep your elbows as far forward as is comfortable. Gently push your wrists together. This should give you a strong stretching sensation in your wrists. Rock 4-10 times.

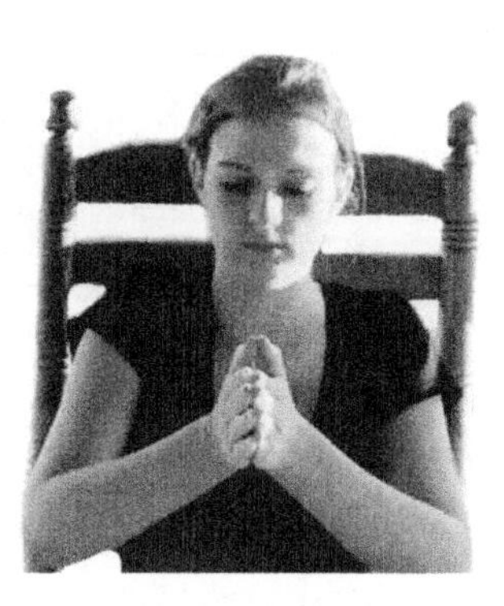

**B. Hold your hands together and tight against the front of your chest. Your fingers should be pointing straight out in front of you. Keep your elbows as far forward as is comfortable. Gently push your wrists together.
Rock 4-10 times.**

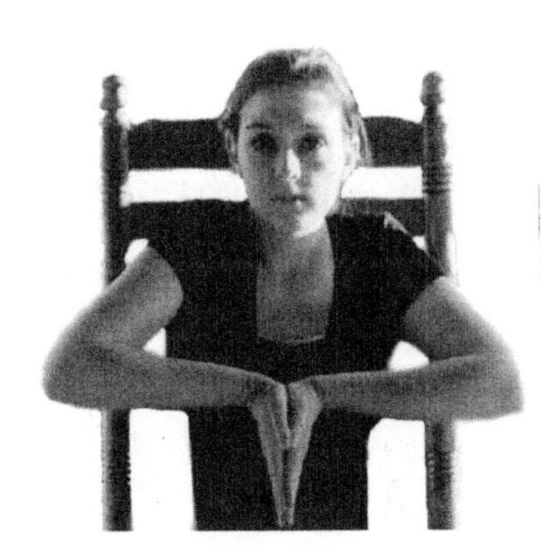

C. Hold your hands together and tight against the front of your chest with your fingers pointing straight down. Keep your elbows as far forward as possible. Gently push your wrists together. Rock 4-10 times.

27 Knees Up And Out

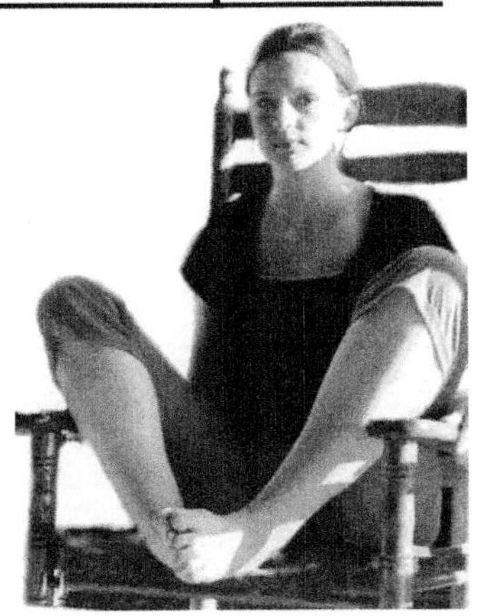

Sit straight up and place your heels on the front middle of the seat. Let the sides of your shins lean out against the armrests. Use your middle body (core) muscles to rock. Rock 4-10 times.

28 Knees Up And In

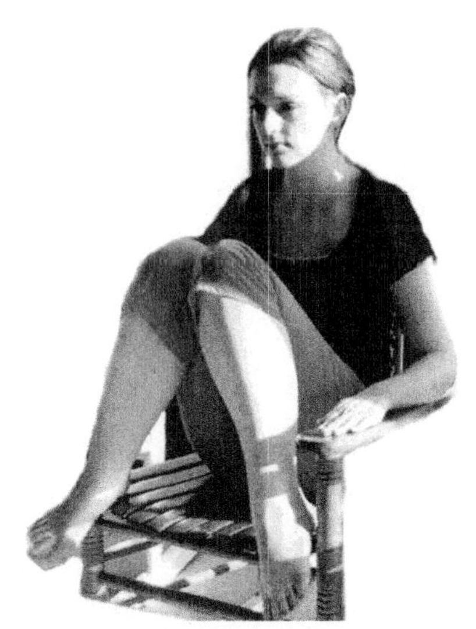

Sit straight up and place your heels on the middle of the seat. Move your feet sideways along the seat front towards the front legs as much as you can. Let your knees touch each other if possible. Use your middle body (core) muscles to rock. Rock 4-10 times.

Chapter 14

Rocking Chair Free Weights Exercises

Be patient as you progress physically. Avoid using too much weight - you may strain a muscle. The following exercises are to be performed using light weights. Hand weights should be used as such: 1-3 pounds for women and 3-5 pounds for men. Please resist the temptation to use heavier weights. Heavy weights have a reputation for causing muscle strain problems.

29 Biceps Curls With Weights

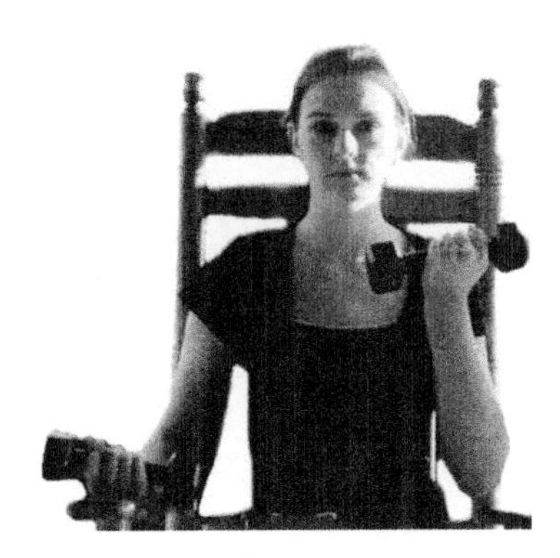

Hold the weights and place both arms on the armrests with your elbows against the back legs of the chair. Raise your arms slightly above the armrests with your hands level and palms up. Flex your left hand up to the front of your left shoulder and then return your hand to the armrest. Alternate your left hand and right hand with each rock. Rock 4-10 times.

Intense 90s: Rotate your hands: thumbs in, thumbs up, and then thumbs outwards.

30 Overhead Presses

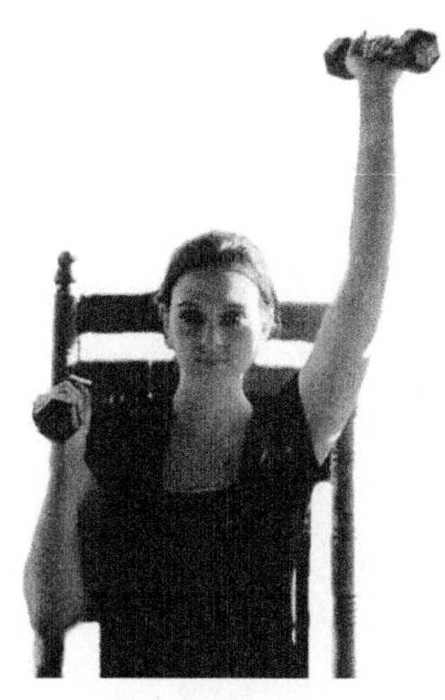

Hold the weights at the tops of your shoulders, neck high and with thumbs pointing backwards.

A. Extend your left arm straight up and then return the weight to neck high.

C. Repeat, raising your right arm. Alternate raising one hand at a time. Rock 4-10 times.

Intense 90s: Rotate your hands, thumbs in, thumbs forward, thumbs backwards.

31 Tilting With Weights

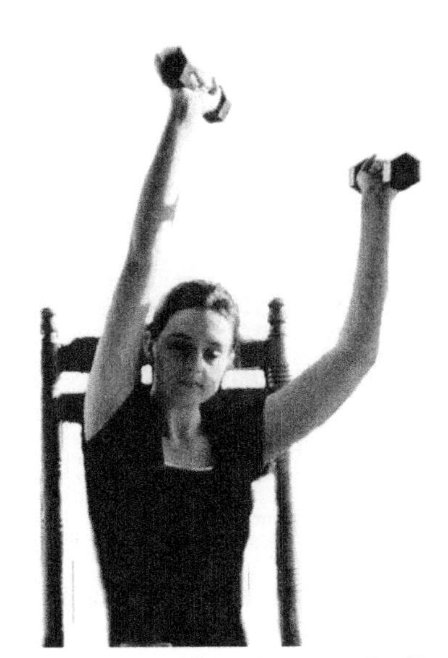

Hold the weights straight up to the sky and tilt from side-to-side.

Rock 4-10 times.

32 Hand Circles With Weights

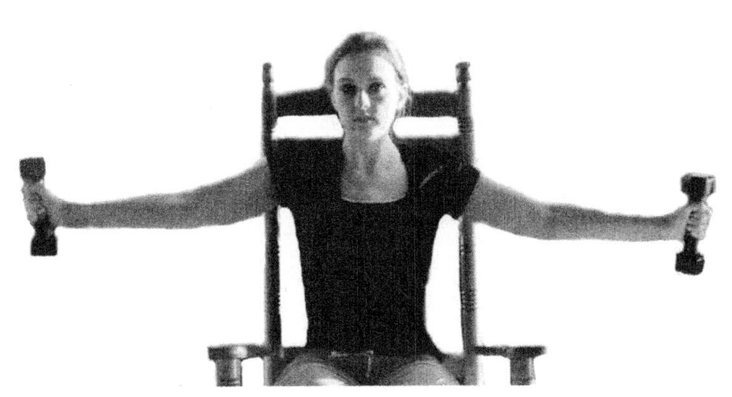

A. Hold the weights straight out to your sides and circle your arms forward.

Rock 4-10 times

B. Circle your arms backwards. Rock 4-10 times.

Intense 90s: While circling, rotate your hands; thumbs down, thumbs forward, thumbs up, and then thumbs backwards.

33 Shoulder Shrugs With Weights

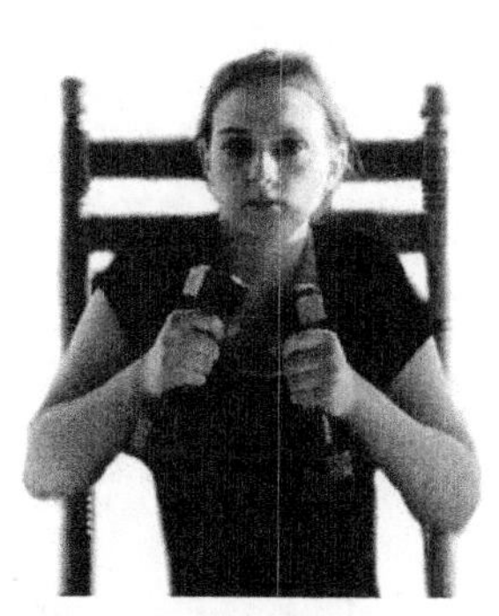

Relax your shoulders. Hold the weights with your elbows bent. Keep your elbows close to your body.

A. Shrug your shoulders forward in a circling motion. Rock 4-10 times.

B. Shrug your shoulders backwards in a cycling motion. Rock 4-10 times.

Intense 90s: Rotate your hands, thumbs in, thumbs upward, and thumbs outward.

34 Weights Above Your Head - 90s

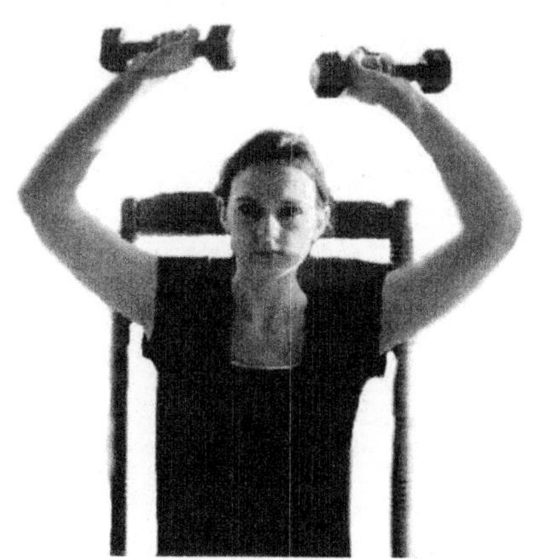

Raise both hands directly above your head. Stay in that position.

Do the 90s; thumbs facing forward, thumbs in, and thumbs facing backwards. Rock 4-10 times.

35 Triceps Lift

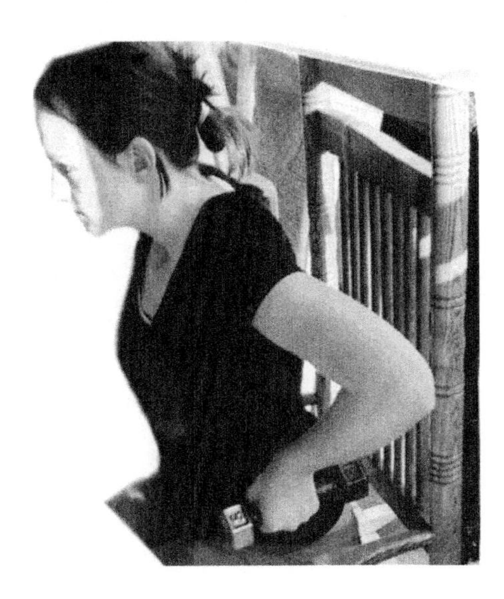

Hold the weights. Hold your elbows to the sides of the back legs of the rocking chair. With your thumbs facing downward, push your elbows back as far as is comfortable and then lift and lower your elbows with an up and down motion. Rock 4-10 times.

Intense 90s: Rotate your hands: thumbs facing backwards, thumbs facing in, thumbs facing forward, then thumbs facing outward.

36 Arms And Wrists 90s

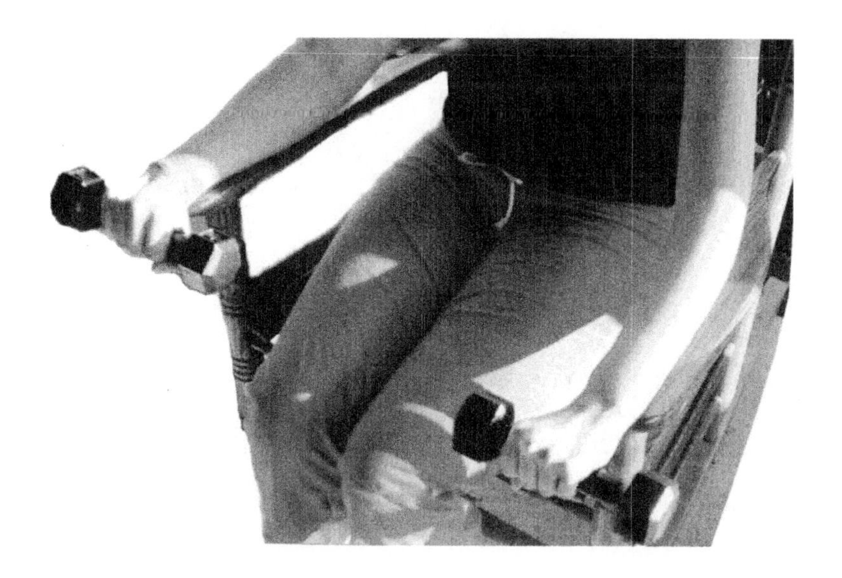

Hold both arms just above the armrests, while holding the weights.

Do the 90s with your hands in this position.

A. Turn your hands so that your thumbs are facing downward.

Rock 4-10 times.

B. Turn your hands so that your thumbs are faces inward.

Rock 4-10 times.

C. Turn your thumbs facing up.

Rock 4-10 times.

D. Turn your thumbs outward.

Rock 4-10 times.

37 Biceps Tense With Weights

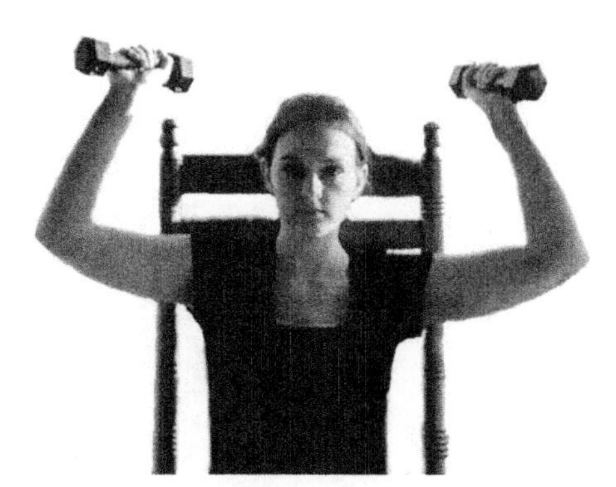

Raise the weights above your head, keeping your upper arms level to the ground. Keep your elbows bent and pointing out toward your sides. Your forearms are extended straight up. Do the 90s with your hands: turn your hands so that your thumbs face backwards, and then forward. Rock 4-10 times.

38 Hand Weight Crossovers

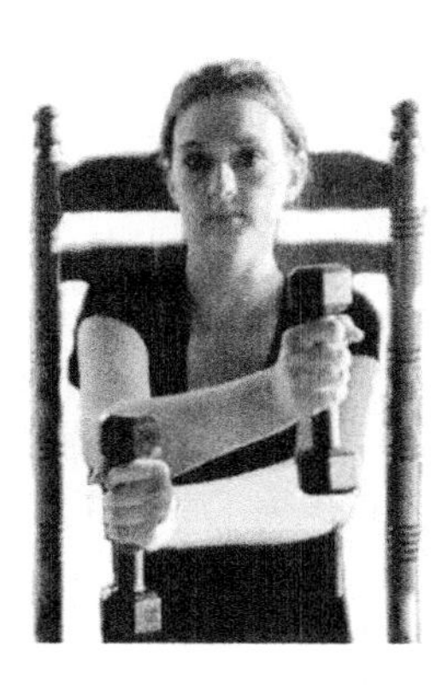

Hold the hand weights out, chest high, at a 45-degree angle. Swing your arms across your knees so that your right hand goes over to your left side and your left hand goes to your right. On each repetition, vary from right hand on top to left hand on top. Rock 4-10 times.

Intense 90s: Rotate your hands: thumbs inward, thumbs upward and then thumbs outward.

39 Nine Pack With One Weight

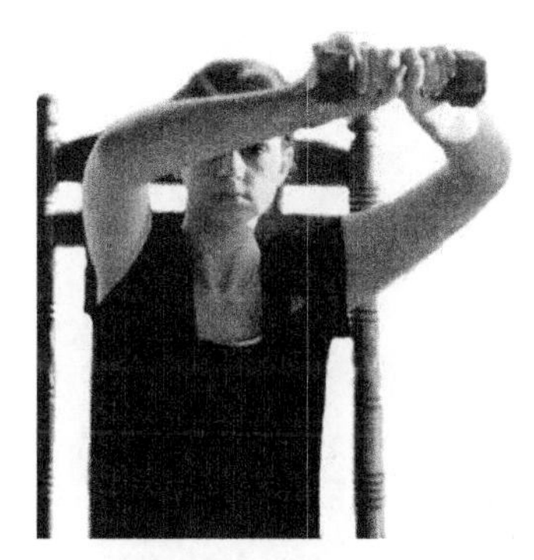

Hold one weight with both hands and with your elbows slightly bent.

1. **Hold the weight at arms length and at eye level. A. Stretch up to your left. Rock 4-10 times.**

   B. Stretch up to your right. Rock 4-10 times.

   C. Stretch straight ahead. Rock 4-10 times.

2. **Hold the weight at arms length and well above your forehead. A. Stretch up to your left. Rock 4-10 times.**

   B. Stretch up to your right. Rock 4-10 times.

   C. Stretch straight ahead. Rock 4-10 times.

3. **Hold the weight at arms length well above and slightly behind your head.**

4. **A. Stretch up to your left. Rock 4-10 times.**

   B. Stretch up to your right. Rock 4-10 times.

   C. Stretch straight up. Rock 4-10 times.

 # 40 Steering Wheel

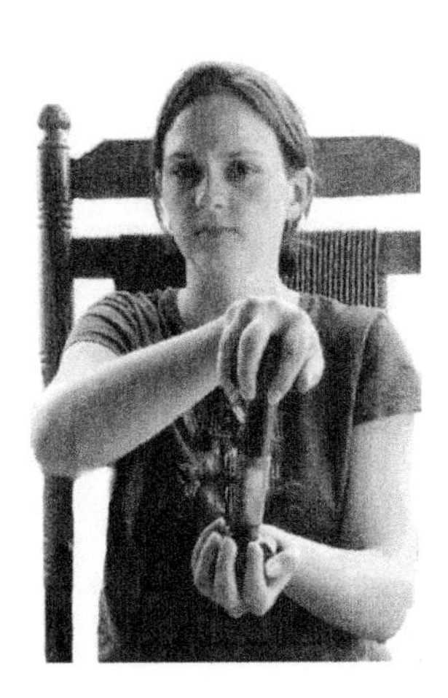

Hold one weight in both hands. Imagine you're driving up and down mountain roads.

A. Turn the weight by lowering your left hand and raising your right. Rock 4-10 times.

B. Lower your right hand and raise your left. Rock 4-10 times.

C. Alternate these positions while rocking. Rock 4-10 times.

<u>#41 Milk Shake</u>

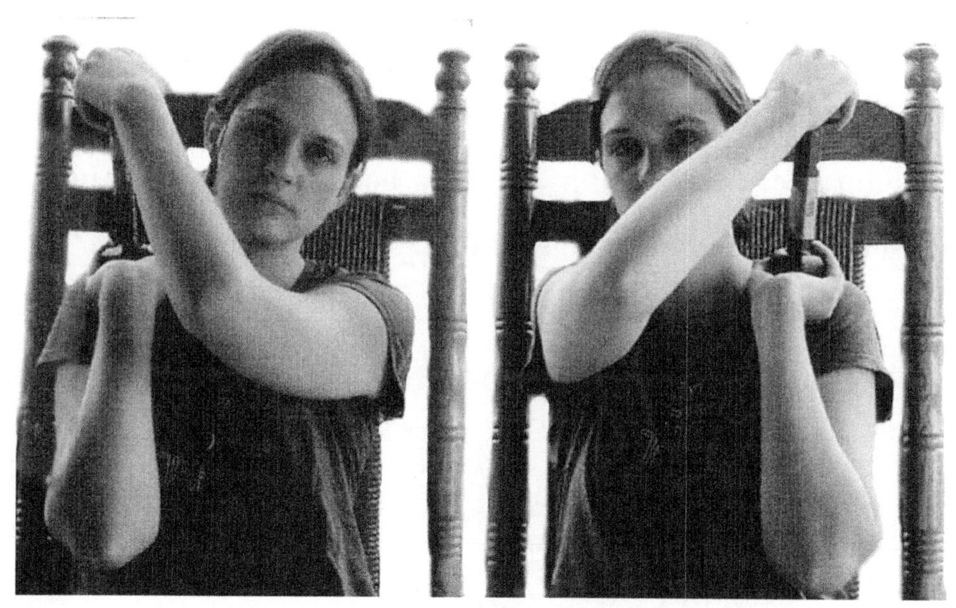

41a	**41b**
Hold the weight over your Right shoulder.	**Hold the weight over your Left shoulder.**

Your knuckles should touch your shoulder each time. Rock, while alternating the weight back and forth from left to right. Rock 4-10 times.

Chapter 15

Rocking Chair Resistance Cord Exercises

The resistance exercises use a cord, band, or tubing to simulate bow and arrow motions.

42 Bow And Arrow To Left Side

Grasp the resistance cord and hold it like it's a bow and arrow. Think of your left hand as holding the bow and your right hand as holding the strings.

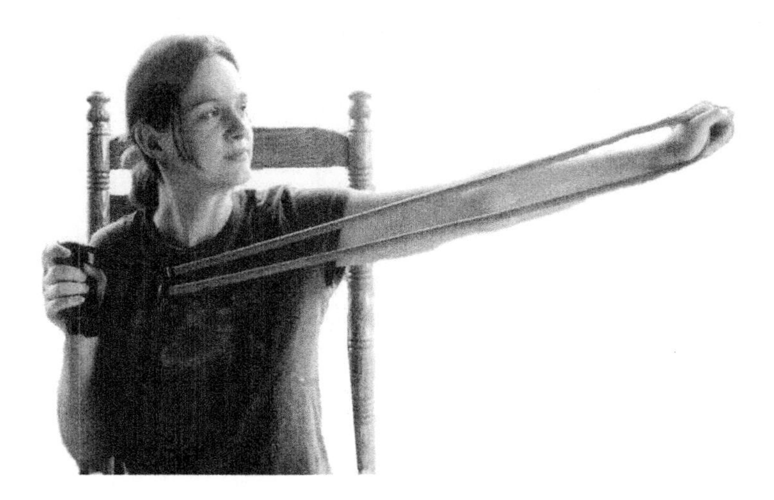

A. Point your left hand (bow) directly towards your left side. Stretch the cord and rock 4-10 times.

B. Gradually move your left hand forward, with two 45-degree moves, until you get to directly forward.
Rock 4-10 times in each 45-degree position.

 # 43 Bow And Arrow To Right Side

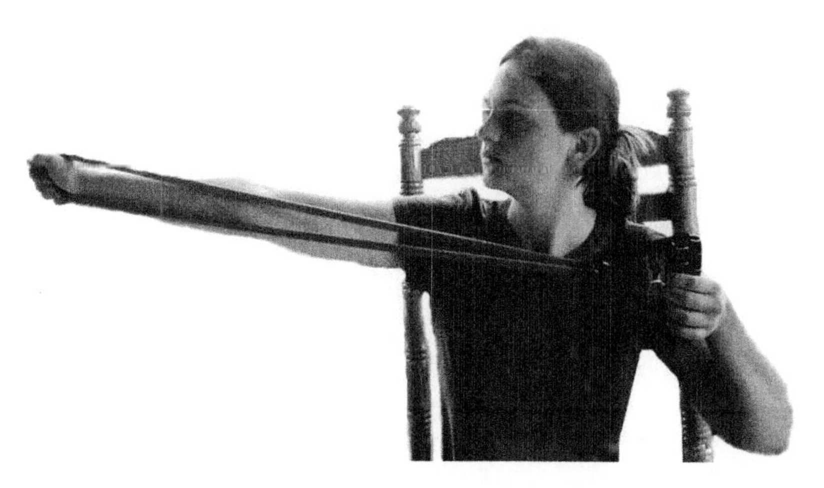

Switch hands, your right hand now holding the bow and your left hand holding the strings.

A. Point your right hand (bow) directly towards your right side.
Stretch the cord.
Rock 4-10 times.

B. Gradually move your right hand forward, with two 45-degree moves, until you get to directly forward.
Rock 4-10 times in each 45-degree position.

44 Bow And Arrow To Right At 45-Degrees

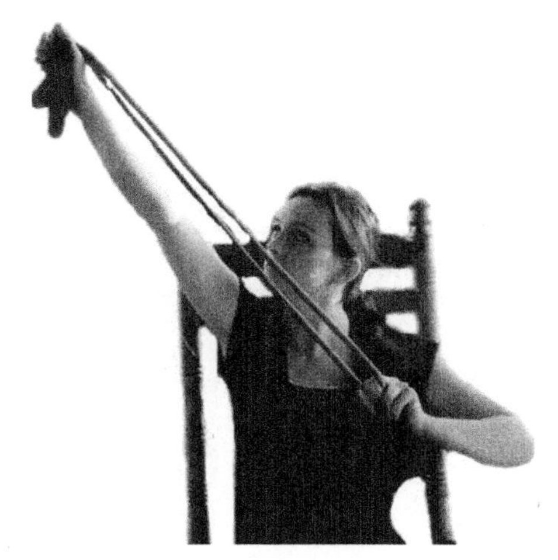

A. Point your right hand (bow) directly towards your right side and up at a 45-degree angle.
Stretch the cord and rock 4-10 times.

B. Keep your right hand up at a 45-degree angle.
Gradually move your right hand forward, with two 45 degree moves, until you get to directly forward.
Rock 4-10 times in each 45-degree position.

45 Bow And Arrow Up To left At 45-Degrees

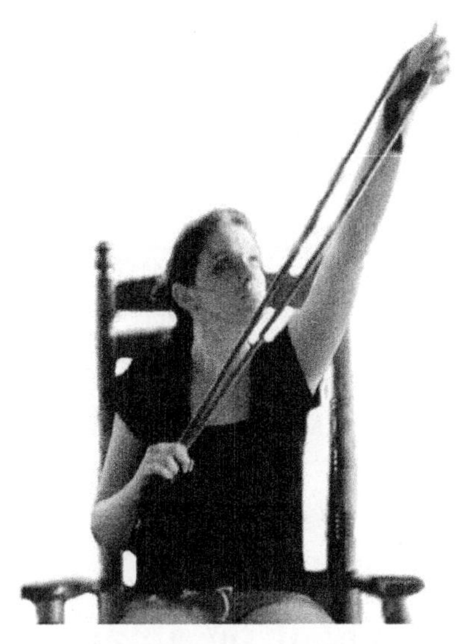

A. Point your left hand (bow) directly towards your left side and up at a 45-degree angle. Stretch the cord and rock 4-10 times.

B. Keep your left hand up at the 45-degree angle. Gradually move your left hand forward, with two 45 degree moves, until you get to directly forward.
Rock 4-10 times in each 45-degree position.

46 Bow And Arrow Straight Up And Down

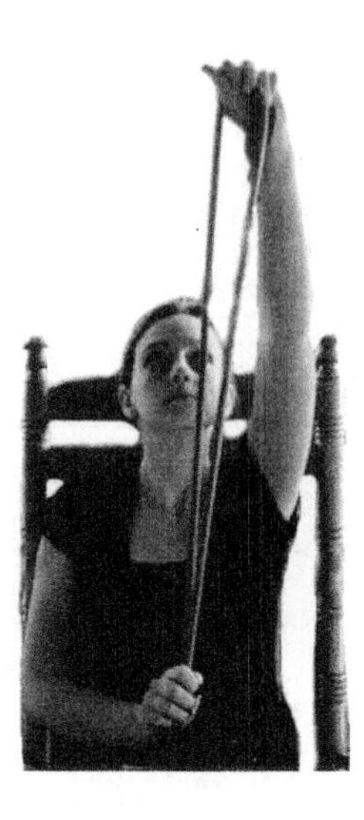

A. Raise your left hand (bow) straight up in the air and just in front of your face.

Your right hand should be almost on your lap. Stretch the cord.

Rock 4-10 times.

B. Raise your right hand (bow) straight up in the air and just in front of your face.

Your left hand should be almost on your lap. Stretch the cord.

Rock 4-10 times.

Chapter 16

Rocking Chair Breathing Exercises

47 Deep Breathing Exercises

The Rocking Chair Breathing Exercises need a little concentration and may be a little difficult to master. The rhythm of the exercises should be achievable in time.

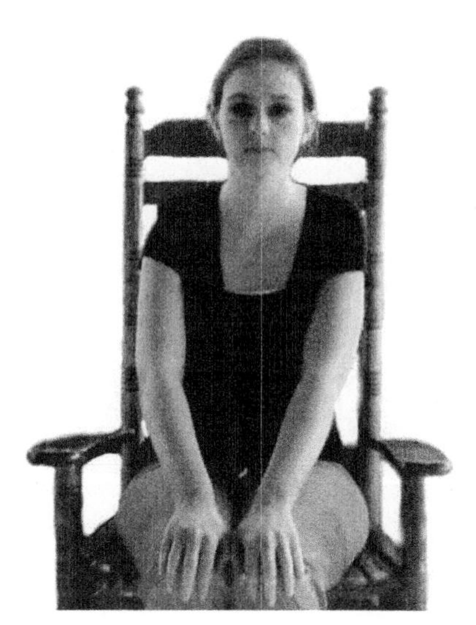

1. Inhale:

A. Inhale deeply through your nose, pushing your abdominal area out to allow air to enter the lower parts of your lungs. Rock one time.

B. Continue by breathing air into your chest and filling the upper parts of your lungs. Rock one time.

2. Hold Your Breath And Rock 2 Times.

3. Exhale:

A. **Pull your abdominal area in and up. Exhale the air from your lower parts of your lungs through your mouth. Rock one time.**

B. **Continue exhaling the air from the upper parts of your lungs. Rock one time. Relax for 2 rocks. Repeat the process 3 or more times.**

Precaution - Do not attempt to deep breathe for long sessions until you get accustomed to deep breathing. You may end up with hard internal muscle spasms.

#48 Lung Expansions

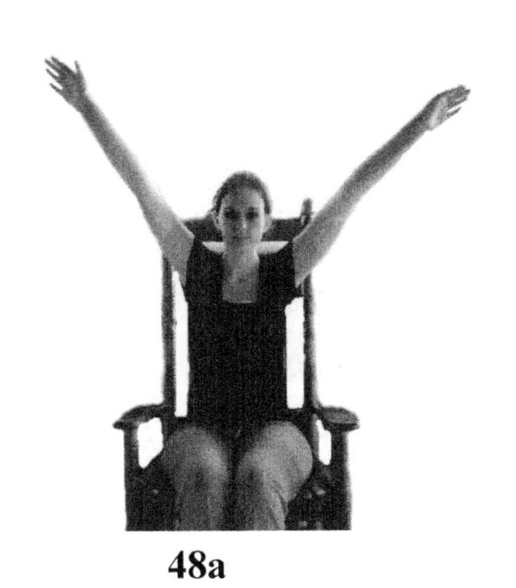

48a

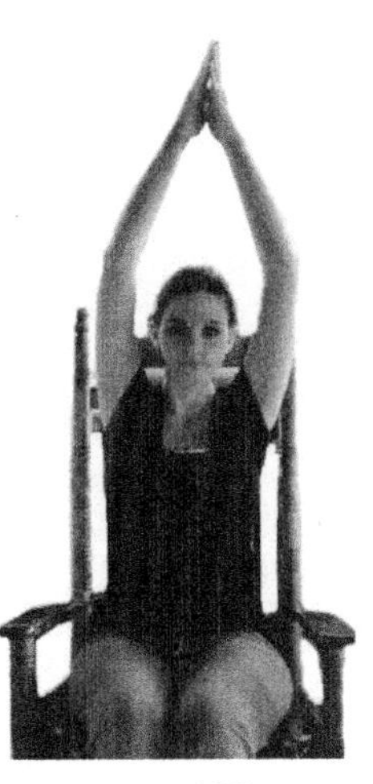

48b

Breathe deeply as you rock. Starting with your hands in your lap, raise your arms to your sides' 48a and then over your head 48b. Return your hands to your lap and repeat the exercise.

Rock and breathe as in exercise # 47.

Chapter 17

Neck Stretches

49 Neck Stretches

Stand up and face the rocking chair. Do not rock the chair during this exercise - you're only using the chair for balance and as a support in case you get dizzy. Place your hands flat on top of the front of the seat, one hand next to each of the front legs. Let your head hang directly down between your elbows in a relaxed manner, allowing a free-flowing movement of your neck muscles. Do not tighten up your neck muscles in order to 'muscle' your way through the exercises - it will work against you and the muscles won't stretch. Think of a cat swinging at a ball on a string. Always keep your head lower than your neck. You really get a good muscle stretch using your head as a weight. Relax and let your neck stretch.

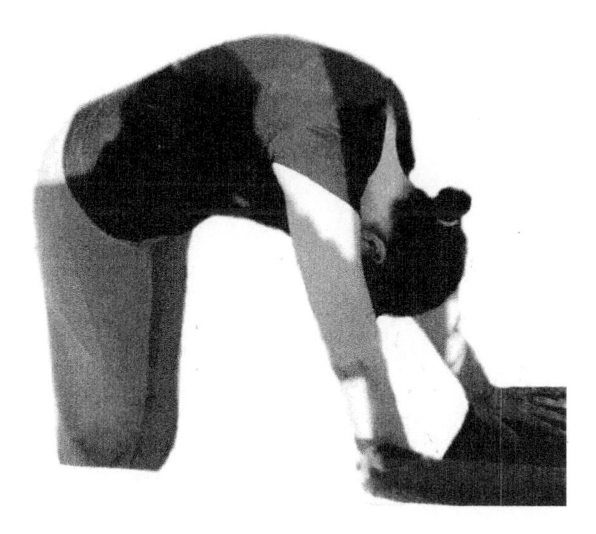

A. Relax your neck muscles and nod your head 'yes' 4-10 times.

B. Twist your head 'no' 4-10 times. The 'no' motion appears to create the most effective neck stretches.

C. Roll your neck back and forth in a neck-roll pattern, left and then right 4-10 times.

D. Move your head slowly from side-to-side like you're ringing a bell 4-10 times.

E. Repeat as desired.

Chapter 18

Target Areas Of Rocking Chair Exercises

Target area	Exercise number(s) 1-28	29-48
Abdominal muscles	All	All
Achilles Tendons	All	All
Ankles	All - Note A	All
Arms	All	29-46, 48
(armpits)	4, 6-10, 17-19, 25 especially 7	30-32, 34-35, 37-46, 48
Biceps	3, 17-19 especially 23	29-46, 48, especially 29
Breathing	All	All especially 47-48
Buns (buttocks)	All	All
Calves	All	All
Core muscles	All	All
Ears	22	
Elbows	2-12, 17-20, 23-26	29-46, 48 especially 40, 41
Feet	All - Note A	All
Fingers	2, 3 Note B	
Forearms	2, 3, 17-19 Note B	29-46, 48
Hands	2, 3 Note B	29-46, 48

Hips	**All**	**All**
Jowls	**21 and 21 Intense**	
Knees	**All especially 13-16 and 27-28**	

Target area	**Exercise number(s) 1-28**	**29-48**
Waist	**All**	**All**
Neck	**21and 21 Intense**	
Oblique muscles	**All**	**All**
Pectoral muscles	**All especially 6, 7, 40, 41**	**All**
Ribs	**4-12, 17-20, 23-24**	**30-35, 38-46, 48**
Saddle bags	**All**	**All**
Shoulders	**4-12, 17-20, 23-25**	**29-46, 48 especially 40, 41**
Thighs-inner	**All**	**All**
Thighs-outer	**All**	**All**
Trapezius muscles	**All**	**All especially 40,41**
Triceps	**5,7-12, 17-19, 24-25,**	**30-46, 48 especially**
Wrists	**2, 3, 26**	**29-32, 34-41**

Note A: All provided the person is barefoot or is in soft socks or similar flexible footwear.

Note B: Provided the person alternates their feet back and forth from duck-foot to pigeon-toed with each rock.

Have a Great Forever. I'd like to leave you with a few positive thoughts for each day. (For Sunday - remember football's 'Super' Sunday).

Brighten the World with your Positive Response

How are you?

"M" is for Monday	**"Marvelous"**
"T" is for Tuesday	**"Terrific"**
"W" is for Wednesday	**"Wonderful"**
"T" is for Thursday	**"Tremendous"**
"F" is for Friday	**"Fabulous"**
"S" is for Saturday	**"Sensational"**
"S" is for Sunday	**"Super"**

Leave people with an eternal blessing - "Have a Great Forever."

Printed in Great Britain
by Amazon

37886361R00072